This book has been sponsored by Ethicon Endo-Surgery (Europe) GmbH and Johnson & Johnson MEDICAL GmbH, Norderstedt, Germany. The authors are responsible for the content of the publication. Information provided in this book is offered in good faith as an educational tool for health care professionals. The information has been thoroughly reviewed and is believed to be useful and accurate at the time of its publication, but is offered without warranty of any kind. The authors and the sponsors shall not be responsible for any loss or damage arising from its use.

Operation Primer

STAPLED TRANSANAL RECTAL RESECTION (STARR)

with Contour® Transtar™
Curved Cutter Stapler Procedure Set

Editors

Marc Immenroth
Thorsten Berg
Jürgen Brenner

Authors

STARR Pioneers

assisted by

Ann-Katrin Güler
Monika Udy-Vejmelkova
Birgit Wahl
Ute Stefani Haaga

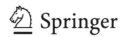 Springer

Authors

Eloy Espin Basany, M.D., Hospital Universitari Vall d'Hebron,
Pg. Vall D'Hebron, 119-129, 08035 Barcelona, Spain

Fabrice Corbisier, M.D., CH Notre-Dame et Reine Fabiola, Site Clinique Notre-Dame,
Grand-rue 3, 6000 Charleroi, Belgium

Franc Hetzer, M.D., Kantonsspital St. Gallen,
Rorschacher Strasse 95, 9007 St. Gallen, Switzerland

David Jayne, M.D., St. James's University Hospital, Academic Surgical Unit,
Level 8 Clinical Sciences Bldg, St. James's University Hospital, Leeds LS9 7TF, UK

Leonardo Lenisa, M.D., Casa di Cura San Pio X, Dept. Surgery,
Via F. Nava, 31, 20159 Milano, Italy

Karen Nugent, M.D., Southampton General Hospital,
Tremona Road, Southampton, S016 6YD, UK

François Pigot, M.D., Bagatelle – Maison de Santé Protestante de Bordeaux,
201, rue Robespierre, B.p. 48, 33401 Talence Cedex, France

Roland Scherer, M.D., Krankenhaus Waldfriede,
Argentinische Allee 40, 14163 Berlin, Germany

Oliver Schwandner, M.D., Caritas Krankenhaus St. Josef,
Landshuter Str. 65, 93053 Regensburg, Germany

Angelo Stuto, M.D., Ospedale S. Maria degli Angeli,
Via Montereale, 24, 33170 Pordenone, Italy

Jean-Jacques Tuech, M.D., PhD, CHU Hopitaux de Rouen, Chirurgie Digestive,
1, rue de Germont, 76031 Rouen cedex, France

Editors

Marc Immenroth, PhD, European Clinical Studies Manager, Ethicon Endo-Surgery (Europe) GmbH,
Hummelsbütteler Steindamm 71, 22851 Norderstedt, Germany

Thorsten Berg, M.D., Director Outcomes Research, Johnson & Johnson Medical Pty Ltd,
1–5 Khartoum Road, North Ryde, NSW 2113, Australia

Jürgen Brenner, M.D., Director European Surgical Institute, a division of Johnson & Johnson MEDICAL GmbH,
Hummelsbütteler Steindamm 71, 22851 Norderstedt, Germany

ISBN 978-3-540-92958-1 Stapled Transanal Rectal Resection (STARR) with Contour® Transtar™ Curved Cutter Stapler Procedure Set

Bibliografische Information der Deutschen Bibliothek
The Deutsche Bibliothek lists this publication in Deutsche Nationalbibliographie;
detailed bibliographic data are available in the internet at http://dnb.ddb.de.

First published in Germany in 2009 by Springer Medizin Verlag
springer.com

SPIN 12586769
Layout and typesetting: Dr. Carl GmbH, Stuttgart, Germany
Printing: Stürtz GmbH, Würzburg, Germany

18/5135/DK – 5 4 3 2 1 0

Editors' preface

The idea for the Operation Primer originated in a scientific study entitled "Mental Training in Surgical Education" that formed part of a collaborative project between the surgical department of the University of Cologne, the Institute of Sports and Sport Sciences of the University of Heidelberg and the European Surgical Institute (ESI) in Norderstedt.

The aim of the study was to evaluate the effect of mental training, which has been used successfully in top-class sports for decades, on surgical training. However, in order for mental training to be applied to surgery, it first had to undergo modification. In the course of this modification, the first Operation Primer was produced, the layout of which was largely adopted for the final version presented here.

Over several years the design of the Operation Primer was optimized and applied to other operations. At the same time, a team of authors was found who could transform the concept into a series of practical surgical primers. For this Operation Primer our first and very special thanks go to the STARR Pioneers, without whom it would not have been possible even to begin to think of converting our ideas into reality.

The text of the Operation Primer is fully comprehensible only when used in conjunction with the accompanying photographs. We would like to thank Federico Pengo, who made and edited the pictures featured in the Operation Primer.

Reality often requires an abstraction in order to make certain situations clearer. This was the reason for including line drawings throughout the Operation Primer. These diagrams were produced by Thomas Heller, whom we gratefully acknowledge.

Our concept of practical surgical primers will become a reality through Dr. Carl GmbH and Springer Medizin Verlag Heidelberg.

The Operation Primer series will be produced with the aim of describing the various operations in the simplest possible manner, but without over-simplifying. Although most time has been spent on the establishment of the scientific basis behind the operations, the main focus has always been on the practical relevance of the primers.

With this Operation Primer we hope we have met our own as well as the readers' highest expectations.

The Editors   May 2009

Authors' preface

How did the STARR idea come about? The experience with stapled prolapsectomy for the treatment of hemorrhoids led to the idea that resection of internal mucosal prolapse could improve rectal evacuation. Based on this idea, and with evidence gained from cadaver studies, Antonio Longo proposed the full-thickness resection of the lower rectum to treat Obstructed Defecation Syndrome (ODS) in patients with rectocele and rectal intussusception. Antonio Longo made the first presentation of this novel technique during a workshop held in Vienna, at the St. Elizabeth Hospital, in December 2000.

The aim of the STARR procedure is to produce a full-thickness rectal resection (Stapled Transanal Rectal Resection). The initial STARR technique included the use of two PPH01 staplers, as at that time there were no dedicated devices for the STARR procedure. Although the functional results achieved with PPH01 staplers were good, there was room for enhancement of the stapler to give the surgeon a degree of flexibility to improve the anatomical correction necessary for best functional outcome.

For this reason a new stapler was devised specifically for use in STARR: a curved cutting stapler with a 30-mm staple line. Ethicon Endo-Surgery has marketed this new device under the name Contour® Transtar™ Curved Cutter Stapler Procedure Set.

Since there was no common understanding of ODS and its most appropriate diagnostic and therapeutic treatment options at that time, the STARR Pioneers group was formed in the fall of 2006. Who or what exactly is a Pioneer? A pioneer is a person who opens up new areas of thought, research and development and becomes instrumental in the growth of something, especially in its early stages.

The STARR Pioneers are a team of 11 colorectal experts from seven European countries. The primary objectives of the STARR Pioneers were to obtain alignment and reach consensus regarding ODS and STARR, to discuss STARR as the treatment option of choice for ODS patients, to create a European network around ODS and STARR, and finally to increase the quality of life for patients.

To date, the group has defined the patient selection criteria, written the STARR Algorithm (Schwandner et al., 2008), fine-tuned procedure steps, established a training protocol, trained and proctored more than 350 European surgeons, and completed the Contour® Transtar™ Stapler feasibility study, which has been accepted for publication (Lenisa et al., in press). In addition, the group presented STARR workshops during the 2nd World Congress of Coloproctology and Pelvic Diseases in Rome in June 2007, during the 2007 Colorectal Congress in St. Gallen, Switzerland, and during the 2008 European Society of Coloproctology Congress in Nantes.

This Operation Primer is a tool to aid in comprehending the STARR procedure performed with Contour® Transtar™ Stapler, including tips and tricks and discussion of potential intraoperative complications and how to avoid them. The Primer cannot replace the appropriate training needed for the use of the Contour® Transtar™ Curved Cutter Stapler.

STARR Pioneers   May 2009

Authors

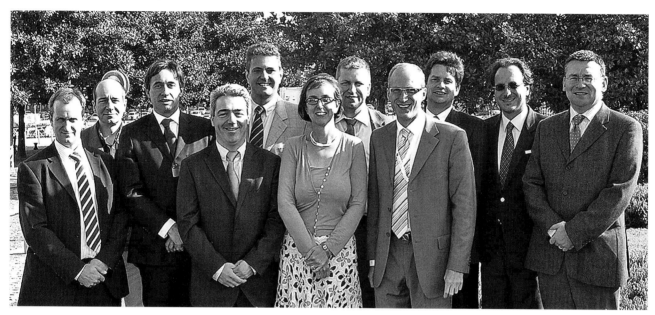

Front row (left to right): Eloy Espin Basany, Karen Nugent, François Pigot
Back row (left to right): David Jayne, Jean-Jacques Tuech, Angelo Stuto, Oliver Schwandner, Roland Scherer, Franc Hetzer, Leonardo Lenisa, Fabrice Corbisier

Eloy Espin Basany, M.D.

– Studied Medicine in Monterrey, Mexico
– 1992–1997 Surgical training at the University Hospital Vall d'Hebron, Barcelona, Spain
– 1999 Doctorate in Medicine at the University of Barcelona, Spain
– Since 1999 Associate Professor and Chief of the Colorectal Surgery Unit of the General Surgery Department at the University Hospital Vall d'Hebron, Barcelona, Spain
– Since 2005 Chief of the Colorectal Surgery Unit of the General Surgery Department at the University Hospital Vall d'Hebron, Barcelona, Spain

Memberships

– 2000 Secretary of Docent Unit of Medicine Faculty at the Autonomous University of Barcelona
– Since 2001 Member of the European Board of Coloproctology (UEMS.EBSQ-Col)
– Since 2006 Examiner at the European Board of Surgical Qualification (EBSQ) Coloproctology Exam
– Since 2008 International Fellow of the American Society of Colon and Rectal Surgeons (ASCRS)

Fabrice Corbisier, M.D.

- Studied Medicine in Louvain en Woluwe, Belgium
- 1986 Doctorate in Medicine at the University of Louvain, Belgium
- 1992 Qualified as General Surgeon
- Since 2001 Head of the Visceral and Digestive Surgery Unit at the Hospital CH Notre-Dame et Reine Fabiola in Charleroi, Belgium

Memberships
- Since 1994 Member of the Royal Belgian Society of Surgery
- Since 2003 Member of the Belgian Section of Colorectal Surgery

Franc Hetzer, M.D.

- Studied Medicine in Zurich, Switzerland
- 1993 Doctorate in Medicine at the University of Zurich, Switzerland
- 2002 Postgraduate Fellowship at the Academic Department of Surgery (Prof. NS Williams, M.D.) at the Royal London Hospital, London, UK
- Since 2005 European Board of Surgical Qualification (EBSQ): Coloproctology
- 2006 Venia legendi of the University of Zurich, Switzerland
- Since 2006 Consultant of the Visceral Surgery and Head of the Coloproctology Department at the Cantonal Hospital of St. Gallen, Switzerland
- Since 2008 Swiss Board of Visceral Surgery

Memberships
- Since 2000 Swiss Board of General Surgery
- Since 2005 Member of the European Expert Panel for SNS
- Since 2005 Expert Referee for British Journal of Surgery
- Since 2007 Examiner at the European Board of Surgical Qualification (EBSQ) Coloproctology Exam
- Since 2008 President of the Swiss Study Group of Sacral Neuromodulation

David Jayne, M.D.

- 1986 Bachelor of Science (BSc) in Anatomy, University of Wales, UK
- 1989 Bachelor of Medicine and Surgery (MB BCh), University of Wales, UK
- 2002 Doctorate in Medicine at the University of Leeds, UK
- Since 2002 Senior Lecturer and Consultant Surgeon, University of Leeds and St. James's University Hospital, UK

Memberships
- Since 1994 Fellow of the Royal College of Surgeons of England
- Since 2004 Clinical Editor of the "International Journal of Robotics & Computer Assisted Surgery"
- Since 2007 Member of the Research and Audit Committee of the Association of Surgeons of Great Britain and Ireland

Leonardo Lenisa, M.D.

– Studied Medicine in Milan, Italy
– 1993 Doctorate in Medicine at the University of Milan, Italy
– Since 1996 Consultant for Colorectal Surgery in the Surgical Unit at the San Pio X Hospital, Milan, Italy
– 1999 Qualified as General Surgeon
– 2002 Master in Colorectal Surgery at the National Cancer Institute of Milan, Italy
– Since 2008 Research Doctorate in Experimental Surgery and Microsurgery at the University of Pavia, Italy

Memberships
– Since 2002 Member of the Italian Association of Hospital Surgeons (ACOI)
– Since 2002 Member of the Italian Society of Coloproctology (SIUCP)
– Since 2006 Member of the European Society of Coloproctology (ESCP)

Karen Nugent, M.D.

– Studied Medicine in Cambridge and London, UK
– 1987 Bachelor of Surgery and Medicine at the University of London, UK
– 1994 Masters in Surgery at the University of London, UK
– 1998 Fellowship of the Royal College of Surgeons (FRCS), Intercollegiate, UK
– Since 1999 Senior Lecturer and Honorary Consultant at the University of Southampton, UK
– Since 2000 Honorary Consultant at the District Hospital in Salisbury, UK
– 2004 Masters in Education, Open University, UK

Memberships
– 2006 Secretary of the Royal Society of Medicine, Coloproctology Section
– Since 2006 Associate Dean Postgraduate Medicine
– 2008 Secretary of the Association of Coloproctology of Great Britain and Ireland

François Pigot, M.D.

– Studied Medicine in Paris, France
– 1985–1991 Learned Medical and Surgical Proctology at the Hôpital Leopold Bellan (Pr Jean Denis), Paris, France
– 1989 Doctorate in Medicine at the University of Paris, France
– 1989 House Physician at the Hôpitaux de Paris, France
– 1989–1991 Senior Registrar in the Hôpitaux de Paris, France
– 1990 University Degree in Medico-Surgical Proctology, Paris, France
– Since 1999 Head of the Coloproctological Medico-Surgical Unit at the Hôpital Bagatelle, Talence Cedex, Bordeaux, France

Memberships
– 1997–2005 Member of the Board of Directors, Société Nationale Française de Coloproctologie (SNFCP)
– 2000–2005 In charge of the National Inter-University Degree in Coloproctology at the SNFCP

Roland Scherer, M.D.

– Studied Medicine in Erlangen, Freiburg and Berlin, Germany
– 1991 Doctorate in Medicine at the University of Freiburg, Germany
– 2006 European Specialist for Coloproctology (EBSQ)
– Since 2006 Medical Director of the Department of Colorectal and Pelvic Floor Surgery at the Hospital Waldfriede, Berlin, Germany
– 2008 Chairman of the European Meeting "Innovations in Coloproctology", Hospital Waldfriede, Berlin, Germany

Oliver Schwandner, M.D.

– Studied Medicine in Würzburg, Germany
– 1996–2006 Residency and Consultant at the Department of Surgery, University Hospital Schleswig-Holstein, Campus Luebeck, Germany
– 1998 Doctorate in Medicine at the University of Würzburg, Germany
– 2002 Qualified as General Surgeon
– 2005 Qualified as Coloproctologist (EBSQ)
– 2006 Qualified as Visceral Surgeon
– Since 2006 Staff Surgeon in the Department of Surgery and Pelvic Floor Center, Caritas-Krankenhaus St. Josef, Regensburg, Germany

Memberships
– Since 1998 Member of the Bavarian Society of Surgeons
– Since 2000 Member of the International Society of University Colon and Rectal Surgeons (ISUCRS)
– Since 2002 Member of the German Society of Surgeons (DGCh)
– Since 2002 Member of the German Society of General and Visceral Surgeons (DGAV)
– Since 2004 Member of the American Society of Colon and Rectal Surgeons (ASCRS)
– Since 2005 Member of the European Society of Coloproctology (ESCP)
– Since 2005 Member of the German Society of Coloproctology (DGK)
– 2006–2008 German Coordinator of the European STARR Registry

Angelo Stuto, M.D.

– Studied Medicine in Florence, Italy
– 1986 Doctorate in Medicine at the University of Florence, Italy
– 1990 Qualified as Pediatric Surgeon
– Since 1998 Coordinator Colorectal Unit (UCP) in Pordenone, Italy
– 1999 Qualified as General Surgeon
– Since 2004 in charge of Colorectal Surgery at the Department of Surgery at the Hospital S. Maria degli Angeli, Pordenone, Italy
– Since 2004 Coordinator and Faculty of the Master in Proctology at Udine University, School of Medicine, Italy
– Since 2006 Head of the Week Surgery Unit at the Hospital S. Maria degli Angeli, Pordenone, Italy

Memberships

– Since 2001 Member of the Board of the Società Italiana Unitaria di Chirurgia Coloproctologica (SIUCP)
– 2003 National Secretary of the SIUCP
– 2007 Incoming President SIUCP

Jean-Jacques Tuech, M.D., PhD

– Studied Medicine in Marseille, France
– 1991–1997 Resident in the Digestive Surgery Department at the University Hospital of Angers, France
– 1997 Doctorate in Medicine at the University of Angers, France
– 1997 Qualified as General Surgeon
– 1997–2001 Fellowship in Digestive Surgery at the University Hospital of Angers, France
– 2000 Qualified as Digestive Surgeon
– 2001 Master in Medical Ethics at the Université René Descartes, Paris, France
– 2001–2003 Staff member in the Surgical Unit of the Anticancer Center in Strasbourg, France
– 2003–2004 Chief of the Digestive Surgery Department of the Hospital in Mulhouse, France
– Since 2004 Staff member in the Department of Digestive Surgery at the University Hospital of Rouen, France
– 2005 PhD in Medical Ethics at the Université René Descartes, Paris, France
– 2005 Habilitation à diriger des recherches (HDR, authorization to conduct research) at the University of Rouen, France
– 2006 Professor in Digestive Surgery
– Since 2006 Professor of Digestive Surgery in the Department of Digestive Surgery at the University Hospital of Rouen, France

Editors

Marc Immenroth, PhD

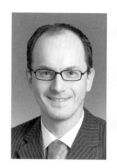

- Studied Psychology (Diploma) and Sports Science (Master) in Heidelberg, Germany
- 1999–2006 Sport Psychologist (including consultant to many German top athletes during their preparation for the World Championships and Olympics) and Industrial Psychologist (including consultant to Lufthansa Inc.)
- 2000 Research Scientist at the University of Greifswald, Germany (Policlinic for Restorative Dentistry and Periodontology)
- 2001–2004 Research Scientist at the University of Heidelberg, Germany (Institute of Sports and Sports Science)
- 2002 Doctorate in Psychology at the University of Heidelberg, Germany
- 2005–2006 Assistant Lecturer at the University of Giessen, Germany (Institute of Sport)
- 2006–2008 Assistant Professor at the University of Greifswald, Germany (Institute of Sport)
- Since 2006 European Clinical Studies Manager at Ethicon Endo-Surgery Europe in Norderstedt, Germany

Focus of Research and Work
- Mental Training in Sport, Surgery and Aviation
- Virtual Reality in Surgical Education
- Coping with Emotion and Stress

Author of many scientific articles and textbooks in psychology, sports science and medicine

Thorsten Berg, M.D.

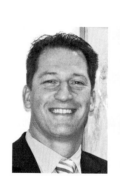

- Studied Medicine in Heidelberg, Germany
- 1996 Intern at the University Hospital, Durban, South Africa
- 1997 Intern at the Surgical Department of the General Hospital, Ludwigshafen, Germany
- 2003 Qualified as General Surgeon
- 2003 Director of Education of European Surgical Institute in Norderstedt, Germany
- 2005 Director of Clinical Development at Ethicon Endo-Surgery Europe in Norderstedt, Germany
- 2006 Senior Manager Health Outcome at Ethicon Endo-Surgery Europe in Norderstedt, Germany
- 2007 Doctorate in Medicine at the University of Heidelberg, Germany
- Since 2008 Director Outcomes Research at Johnson & Johnson Medical in Sydney, Australia

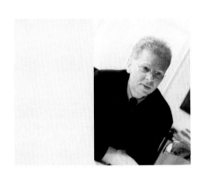

Jürgen Brenner, M.D.

- Studied Medicine in Hamburg, Germany
- 1972 Doctorate in Medicine at the University of Hamburg, Germany
- 1972 Institute for Neuroanatomy, University of Hamburg, Germany
- 1974 Senior Resident at the Department of Surgery of the General Hospital Hamburg-Wandsbek, Germany
- 1981 Medical Director of the Department for Colorectal and Trauma Surgery at St. Adolf Stift Hospital in Reinbek, Germany
- 1987 Director for Surgical Research of Ethicon Inc. in Norderstedt, Germany
- 1989 Director of the European Surgical Institute and Vice President Professional Education Europe at Ethicon Endo-Surgery Europe in Norderstedt, Germany
- 2004 Managing Director at Ethicon Endo-Surgery Germany in Norderstedt, Germany
- Since 2008 Director of the European Surgical Institute in Norderstedt, Germany

Assistants

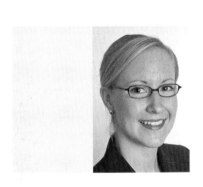

Ann-Katrin Güler

- Studied Medicine in Hamburg, Germany
- Since 2005 doctoral thesis 'Development and evaluation of standardized operation primer for education in minimal invasive surgery' at the University of Hamburg, Germany (Department of General, Thoracic and Visceral Surgery)
- Since 2007 member of the Market Access Department at Ethicon Endo-Surgery Europe in Norderstedt, Germany

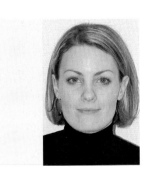

Monika Udy-Vejmelkova

- 2002 Bachelor of Arts in German and Business Administration, Weber State University, Ogden, Utah, USA
- 2004 MBA in International Management, Thunderbird School of Global Management, Glendale, Arizona, USA
- 2004 Customer Care Intern at Cox Communications, Phoenix, Arizona, USA
- 2005 Sales Representative at Johnson & Johnson s.r.o., Prague, Czech Republic
- 2005 Professional Education Specialist at Johnson & Johnson s.r.o., Prague, Czech Republic
- 2007 European Junior Marketing Manager at Ethicon Endo-Surgery Europe, Norderstedt, Germany
- Since 2008 European Marketing Manager at Ethicon Endo-Surgery Europe, Norderstedt, Germany

Birgit Wahl, M.D.

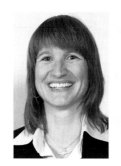

– Studied Medicine in Freiburg, Germany
– 2000–2003 Intern at different Surgical Departments, Germany
– 2003 Doctorate in Medicine at the University of Freiburg, Germany
– 2003–2006 Product Manager at Spitta Publishing House in Balingen, Germany
– Since 2006 Free Medical Writer at Dr. Carl GmbH in Stuttgart, Germany
– Since 2008 certified Medical Journalist, Deutsche Fachjournalisten-Schule in Berlin, Germany

Ute Stefani Haaga, M.D.

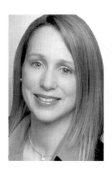

– Studied Medicine in Freiburg, Germany
– 2000–2002 Intern at the Department of Medicine at the University of Erlangen, Germany
– 2001 Doctorate in Medicine at the University of Freiburg, Germany
– Since 2002 Project Manager and Medical Writer at Dr. Carl GmbH in Stuttgart, Germany

Contents

Appendices

Introduction

From an educational point of view, the Operation Primer is somewhat plagiaristic. The layout – and this can be admitted freely – is largely taken over from commonly available cook books. In such books, the ingredients and cooking utensils required to prepare the recipe in question are normally listed first. The most important cooking procedures are then described briefly in the text. Photographs support the written explanations and show what the dish should look like when prepared. Sometimes diagrams and illustrations make individual cooking steps clearer.

Despite these obvious parallels, there is a crucial difference between cook books and the Operation Primer: in the Operation Primer, complicated and complex surgical techniques are described that are intended to help the surgeon and his team perform an operation safely and economically. Ultimately, it always comes down to the patient's welfare. The following must therefore be said early in this introduction:

- The use of the Operation Primer as an aid to operating requires that surgical techniques have first been completely mastered.

- Being alert to possible mistakes is categorically the most important principle when operating; avoiding mistakes is crucial.

As already mentioned in the Editors' preface, the concept of the Operation Primer originated in a scientific study with the title "Mental Training in Surgical Education" that formed part of a collaborative project between the surgical department of the University of Cologne (under Prof. Hans Troidl), the Institute of Sports and Sport Science of the University of Heidelberg, and the European Surgical Institute (ESI) in Norderstedt. Laparoscopic cholecystectomy was the initial focus.

Mental training is derived from top-class sports. This is understood as methodically repeating and consciously imagining actions and movements without actually carrying them out at the same time (cf. Driskell, Copper & Moran, 1994; Feltz & Landers, 1983; Immenroth, 2003; Immenroth, Eberspächer & Hermann, 2008). Scientific involvement with imagining movement has a long tradition in medical and psychological research. As early as 1852, Lotze described how imagining and perceiving movements can lead to a concurrent performance "with quiet movements …" (Lotze, 1852). This phenomenon later became known by the names "Ideomotion" and "Carpenter effect" (Carpenter, 1874).

In the collaborative project, mental training was modified in such a way that it could be employed in the training and further education of young surgeons. In mental training in surgery, surgeons visualize the operation from the inner perspective without performing any actual movements, i.e., they go through the operation step by step in their mind's eye. In the study that was conducted at the ESI, the first Operation Primer was used as the basis for this visualization. In this primer, laparoscopic cholecystectomy was subdivided into individual, clearly depicted steps, the so-called nodal points.

The study evaluated the effect of the mental training on learning laparoscopic cholecystectomy compared with practical training and with a control group. The planning, conduct, and evaluation of the study took seven years (2000–2007), with over 100 surgeons participating.

The results corresponded exactly with the expectations: the mentally trained surgeons improved in a similar degree to those surgeons who received additional practical training on a pelvi trainer simulator (in some subscales even more). Moreover, there was greater improvement in these two groups compared with the control group, which did not receive any additional mental or practical training (cf. in detail, Immenroth, Bürger, Brenner, Nagelschmidt, Eberspächer & Troidl, 2007; Immenroth, Bürger, Brenner, Kemmler, Nagelschmidt, Eberspächer & Troidl, 2005; Immenroth, Eberspächer, Nagelschmidt, Troidl, Bürger, Brenner, Berg, Müller & Kemmler, 2005).

Furthermore, the study included a questionnaire to determine the extent to which the mentally trained surgeons accepted mental training as a teaching method in surgery. Mental training was assessed as very positive by all 34 mentally trained surgeons. The Operation Primer received particular acclaim in the evaluation (cf. in detail, Immenroth et al., 2007):

- 28 surgeons wished to use similar self-made Operation Primers in their daily work.

- 29 surgeons attributed the success of the mental training at least in part to the Operation Primer.

- 30 surgeons wanted to have these Operation Primers as a fixed component of the course at the ESI.

This positive response to the study was the starting point for the production of the present series of Operation Primers.

Prior to publication, the Operation Primer was developed by methodical and didactical means and then adapted to the readers' needs and wishes. This was carried out following a survey of 93 surgeons (interns, resident doctors, assistant medical directors and medical directors) who participated in surgical courses at the ESI. They evaluated in detail the structure and components by means of a questionnaire.

The results of this survey gave important findings on how to optimize the Operation Primer. The sense and representation of the nodal points, the comprehensibility and detail of the text, and the photographs of the operation were highly valued especially by young surgeons (Güler, Immenroth, Berg, Bürger & Gawad, 2006). The comprehensive research undertaken with this Operation Primer series will ensure its overall value to the reader.

Structure and handling of the Operation Primer

In the present series of Operation Primers, an attempt has been made to standardize the described operations as much as possible. This is achieved first by applying the same format to all operational techniques described. Second, operative sequences that are performed identically in all operations are always explained using the same blocks of text. By following a general structure for the description of all operations and by using identical text blocks, it was intended to aid recognition of recurring patterns and their translation into action even for different operations.

The Operation Primer is divided into three chapters, each identified by Roman numerals and different register colors on the margin. The contents of the individual chapters will now be explained.

In **Preparations for the operation,** the instruments for the operation are listed. This is followed by a detailed description of the positioning and shaving of the patient, setting up the equipment, disinfection and sterile draping of the patient. The operative preparation is concluded with a detailed description and picture of how the operating team is to be positioned for the operation in question.

The core of the Operation Primer is the chapter **Nodal points**. This is where the actual sequence of the operation is described in detail. However, prior to this detailed explanation, the term nodal point will be explained briefly. In the Editors' preface and introduction, mental training was mentioned as a form of training used successfully in top-class sports for decades, and this is where the term originates. In sports as in surgery, a nodal point is understood as one of those structural components of movement that are absolutely essential for performing the movement optimally. Nodal points have to be passed through in succession and are characterized by a reduction in the degrees of freedom of action. In mental training they act as orientation points for methodical repetition and conscious imagination of the athletic or operative movement (cf. in detail Immenroth et al., 2008).

For every operation in the Operation Primer series, these nodal points were extracted in a prolonged process by the authors in collaboration with the editors. The nodal points represent the basic structural framework of an operation. Because of their particular relevance and for better orientation, all of the nodal points in the Operation Primer are shown on the left on each double page as a flow chart. The current nodal point is highlighted graphically. An anatomical graphic of the operative site and the instruments required for this nodal point are listed in a box on the right, beside the flow chart.

Below the instrument box, instructions regarding the nodal point are given as briefly as possible. According to Miller (1956), people can best store 7±2 units of information ("Magical number 7"). Therefore, no more than seven single instructions are listed per nodal point, if possible. With regard to the instructions, it should be noted that the change of instruments between the individual nodal points is not described explicitly as a rule; rather, this is apparent through different instruments in the instrument box.

I	Preparations for the operation
II	Nodal points
III	Management of difficult situations, complications and mistakes
	Appendices

Nodal point = term from top-class sports

Nodal points:
1) absolutely essential
2) successive order
3) no degrees of freedom

Flow chart of the sequence of nodal points on each double page

Continuous illustration of the operative site

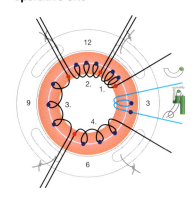

Maximum of 7±2 instructions per nodal point

Danger warnings are pointed out in red!

Alternatives: In small blue print at the end of the nodal point.

Example of an operation note and further details about ODS, patient selection and postoperative management in the appendices

(→ p. 53, III-2) = reference to the 2ⁿᵈ section of chapter III

All sources in the literature are listed in the bibliography

Where necessary, particular moments of danger are pointed out in red.

The described operation sequence is only one way of performing the operation safely and economically, namely the way preferred by the authors. Undoubtedly, a number of other equally valid operation sequences exist. As far as possible, notes on alternative methods are given in small blue print at the end of each nodal point.

In the third chapter, the **Management of difficult situations, complications and mistakes** is described in detail. In general, details on procedure-related complications, e.g., spiraling-in, spiraling-out, dog ears, etc. are given first.

In order to give the Operation Primer even more practical relevance, an example of an operation note is reproduced in the **Appendices**. Besides the operation note, the appendices also contain detailed information about what Obstructed Defecation Syndrome (ODS) is, about patient selection criteria for Stapled Transanal Rectal Resection (STARR), and helpful hints for the postoperative management, as well as the bibliographical references and list of key words.

In order to avoid repetition, reference is made throughout the text to relevant chapters of the Operation Primer, if necessary. To do this, the Roman numeral of the chapter and the number of the corresponding section are shown in parentheses. Referral is made most often to the third chapter where the management of difficult situations, complications and mistakes is described. These references are set off in red letters.

Additionally, it must be pointed out that for better readability of the Operation Primer no bibliographical references at all are given in the text. However, in order to give an overview of the basic and more extensive sources, the entire literature is listed in the bibliography.

Preparations for the operation

Make sure that the following preoperative requirements for Stapled Transanal Rectal Resection (STARR) with Contour® Transtar™ Curved Cutter Stapler Procedure Set have been met:

- The indication for the operation is correct (→ p. 63).

- The patient has given detailed informed written consent.

- A conventional or a magnetic resonance defecography has been performed.

- For elderly female patients a 10-day course of topical estrogen has been administered to minimize the effects of vaginal mucosal atrophy.

- The bowel is prepared appropriately with a cleansing enema.

- The bladder has been emptied by micturition directly before the operation.

- Thromboprophylaxis (low-molecular-weight heparin) has been given as per local practice.

- Single-dose perioperative antibiotic prophylaxis has been given.

Contour® Transtar™ Curved Cutter Stapler Procedure Set

Please be aware that in order to obtain access to the Contour® Transtar™ Curved Cutter Stapler Procedure Set it is necessary to complete a 2-step training program organized by Ethicon Endo-Surgery!

The Contour® Transtar™ Curved Cutter Stapler may be used to approximate tissue in procedures to treat various anorectal wall abnormalities, which could lead to Obstructed Defecation Syndrome (ODS).

Features and benefits

The Contour® Transtar™ Curved Cutter Stapler cuts and staples simultaneously; therefore, no other instruments are necessary to perform the transanal resection.

The unique curved head design facilitates easy placement of the stapler in the rectum due to its conformity to the natural anatomy of the rectum. In comparison to the circular stapler-based approach to STARR, the curved head also allows easier access and enhanced visibility in the narrow anal canal.

Working principles

The Contour® Transtar™ Curved Cutter Stapler is a single-patient-use device. With each firing the device delivers three staggered rows of titanium staples and creates a 30-mm curved transection between the first and second rows of staples. The stapler can be reloaded seven times for a maximum of eight firings in a single procedure.

Equipment

- Contour® Transtar™ Curved Cutter Stapler Procedure Set (STR5G, Ethicon Endo-Surgery):
  - Contour® Transtar™ Curved Cutter Stapler (including 1 cartridge)
  - Circular Anal Dilator
  - Obturator
  - Access Suture Anoscope

- At least 4 Contour® Transtar™ Cartridge Reloads (CR30G, Ethicon Endo-Surgery)

Before using Contour® Transtar™ Curved Cutter Stapler Procedure Set read the instructions for use and make sure that you are familiar with the instrument!

Instruments

- Needle holder

- Suture scissors

- Metzenbaum scissors

- 4 atraumatic forceps

- 6 Mosquito hemostats

- Péan clamp

- 2 Kocher clamps

- Syringe with lubricating jelly

- Compresses

- Swabs

- Sutures:
  - 4 fixation sutures for the Circular Anal Dilator: 0 absorbable, polyfilament
  - 4 parachute sutures for the prolapse: 2–0 absorbable, monofilament
  - Additional parachute sutures, if necessary
  - Traction suture for the opening of the prolapse: 2–0 absorbable, monofilament
  - Marking suture for the end of resection: 2–0 absorbable, polyfilament
  - Hemostatic suture: 3–0 absorbable, monofilament or polyfilament
  - Additional hemostatic sutures, if necessary

- Suction device

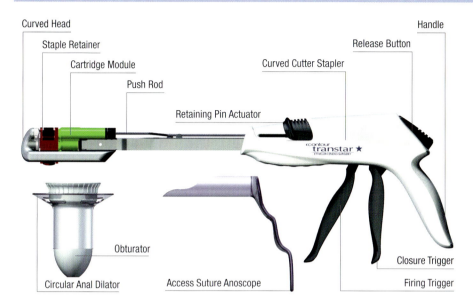

Curved Head
Staple Retainer
Cartridge Module
Push Rod
Retaining Pin Actuator
Curved Cutter Stapler
Handle
Release Button
Obturator
Circular Anal Dilator
Access Suture Anoscope
Closure Trigger
Firing Trigger

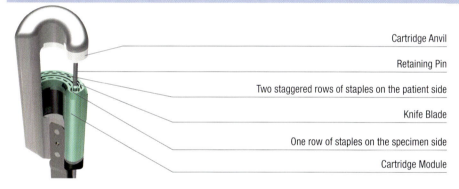

Cartridge Anvil
Retaining Pin
Two staggered rows of staples on the patient side
Knife Blade
One row of staples on the specimen side
Cartridge Module

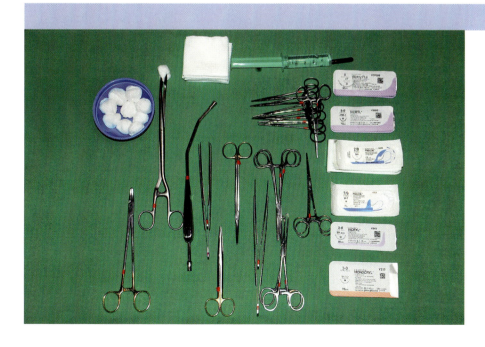

Emptying the bladder

- Place a temporary transurethral catheter.

Positioning of the patient

- Position the patient in lithotomy position with the tip of the coccyx in a line with the end of the operating table.
- Flex the hips to an angle no greater than 90° to 100° in order to avoid injuries to the sciatic plexus.
- Flex the knees to an angle of 90° and position the axis of the lower leg in line with the contralateral shoulder.
- Place both arms at an angle no greater than 70° to the long axis of the body in order to avoid injuries to the axillary nerve.
- Place shoulder supports on both sides to prevent the patient from sliding.
- With men, fix the penis to the abdominal wall with adhesive tape.
- Put the patient into a 30° Trendelenburg position.

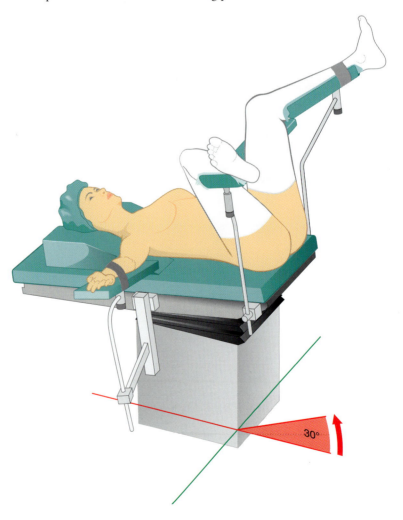

Shaving

- Routine perianal shaving is not mandatory.

Setting up the equipment

- Attach the suction device.

Disinfection

- First disinfect the vagina in women and the scrotum in men with a mounted swab. Then disinfect the anal canal and the distal rectum.

- Disinfect the skin from the pubis in women or the scrotum in men down to the tip of the coccyx and laterally to the inner side of the thighs on both sides. Pay particular attention to careful disinfection of all skin folds.

Sterile draping

- Drape the operating field with adhesive sterile drapes so that it is limited cranially at the level of the mons pubis or the scrotum, caudally below the anus, and laterally parallel to the femoral folds covering them.

- Make sure that the sterile drape allows unlimited access to the anus, the vagina in women, and the perianal and the perineal area.

Positioning of the operating team

Lithotomy and 30° Trendelenburg position

- The surgeon sits at the end of the operating table between the patient's legs.

- The first assistant stands to the left of the surgeon.

- The scrub nurse sits to the right of the surgeon.

Alternative: To increase exposure and therefore to make the procedure easier, it is possible to operate with a second assistant. In this case, the second assistant stands to the right of the surgeon at the level of the patient's left leg.

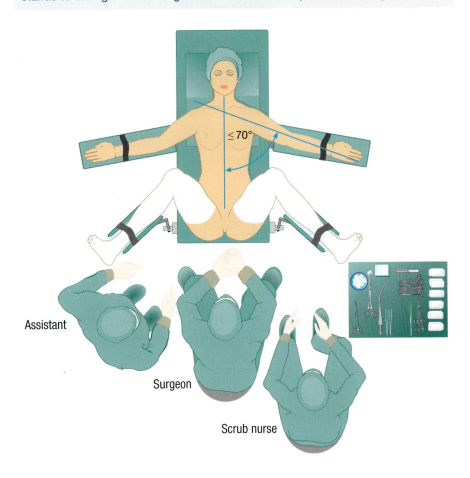

Assistant

Surgeon

Scrub nurse

Nodal points

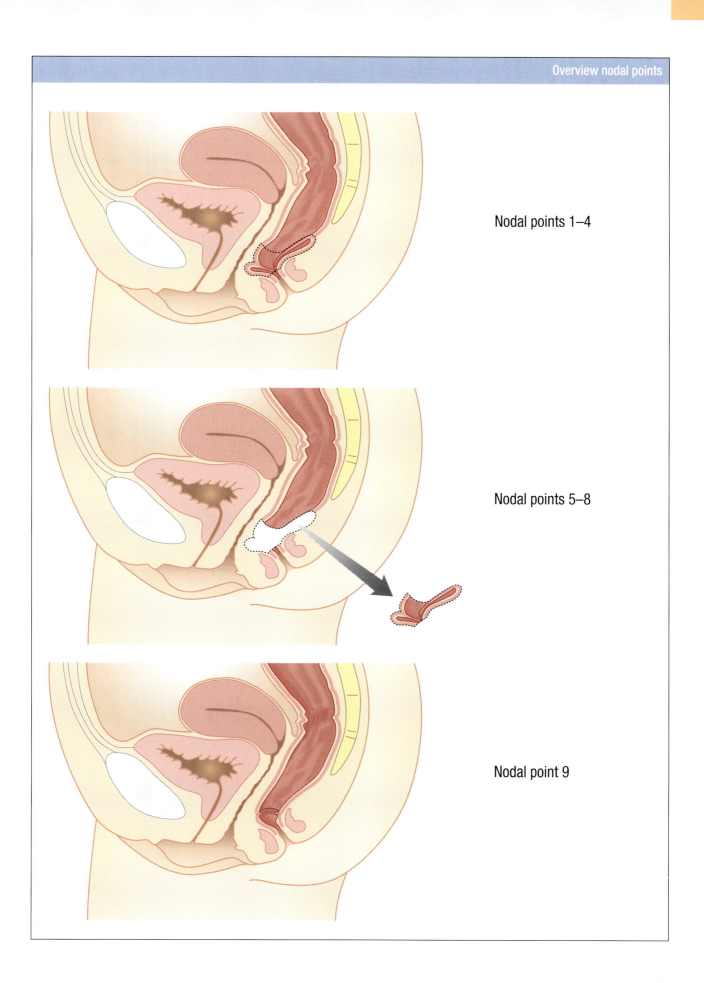

Nodal points 1–4

Nodal points 5–8

Nodal point 9

Nodal point 1 — Introducing the Circular Anal Dilator and exposing the rectal prolapse

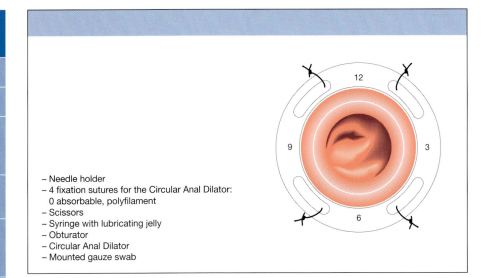

– Needle holder
– 4 fixation sutures for the Circular Anal Dilator:
  0 absorbable, polyfilament
– Scissors
– Syringe with lubricating jelly
– Obturator
– Circular Anal Dilator
– Mounted gauze swab

Pre-place four perianal sutures at approximately 1, 11, 7 and 5 o'clock. They will be used to secure the Circular Anal Dilator.

Lubricate the Obturator. Gently introduce it and stretch the anal sphincter. Dilate the anal sphincter carefully and not too excessively.

Be careful not to dilate the anal sphincter too excessively in order to avoid injury (→ p. 55, III-7c)!

Remove the Obturator.

Fully insert the Circular Anal Dilator together with the Obturator into the anal canal, so that the flange of the dilator is flush with the perineal skin.

Make sure that the perineal skin is not inverted into the anal canal and that the dentate line is protected behind the barrel of the Circular Anal Dilator!

Secure the Circular Anal Dilator with the four perianal sutures and remove the Obturator.

Introduce a dry mounted gauze swab into the rectum. Then slowly pull it out to assess the amount of prolapse, to fold the rectal wall and to expose the apex of the prolapse.

Alternative: Place four perianal sutures after introducing the Circular Anal Dilator and fix the dilator with them.

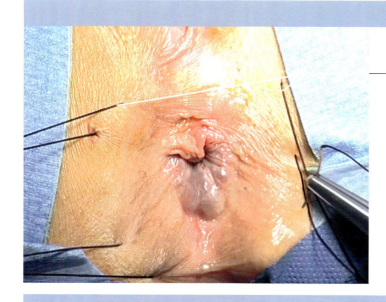

Perianal sutures

Inserting the Circular Anal Dilator with the Obturator

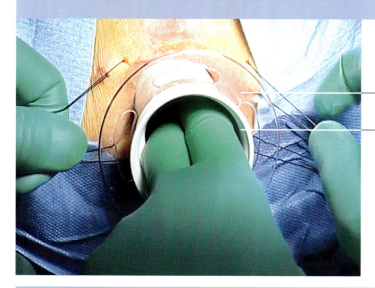

Circular Anal Dilator

Obturator

Pulling out the mounted gauze swab

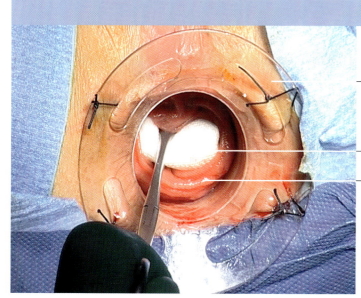

Circular Anal Dilator

Mounted gauze swab

Rectal prolapse

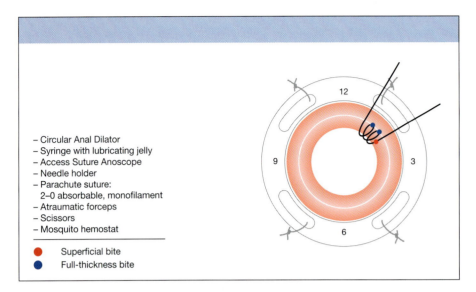

– Circular Anal Dilator
– Syringe with lubricating jelly
– Access Suture Anoscope
– Needle holder
– Parachute suture:
  2–0 absorbable, monofilament
– Atraumatic forceps
– Scissors
– Mosquito hemostat

● Superficial bite
● Full-thickness bite

In order to achieve symmetrical traction of the prolapse around its circumference, several parachute sutures need to be placed.

Lubricate the Access Suture Anoscope. Then insert it into the Circular Anal Dilator with the open window positioned at around 2 o'clock in order not to inadvertently catch tissue from the opposite rectal wall or the vagina in women.

It is important to insert the anoscope into the anal canal before performing the first stitch in order not to inadvertently catch tissue from the opposite rectal wall or the vagina (→ p. 55, III-7a, b)!

Place the first bite of the first parachute suture superficially on top of the prolapse at around 2 o'clock and remove the anoscope.

Position the following two to three full-thickness bites as a running suture counter-clockwise from 2 to 1 o'clock, capturing the apex of the prolapse. Perform these bites deep enough to expose the prolapse and to gain solid traction on it. With the first parachute suture, capture 1–2 cm of the tissue circumferentially.

Tie the suture loosely in order to allow for good traction on the captured tissue.

Make sure to place the full-thickness bites of the parachute suture deep enough to expose the prolapse, and tie the suture loosely to gain good traction on the captured tissue (→ p. 53, III-2)!

Connect the ends of the threads with a Mosquito hemostat and keep the suture under traction.

Alternative: Instead of the Access Suture Anoscope place a mounted gauze swab into the anal canal before performing the first stitch.

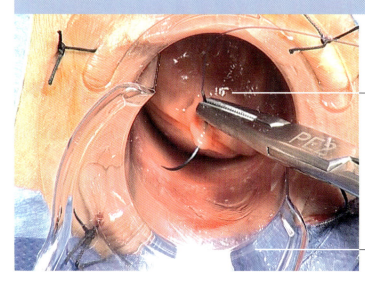

Placing the superficial bite of the first parachute suture

Rectal prolapse

Access Suture Anoscope

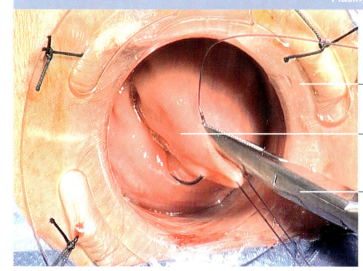

Placing the first full-thickness bite of the first parachute suture

Circular Anal Dilator

Rectal prolapse

Needle holder

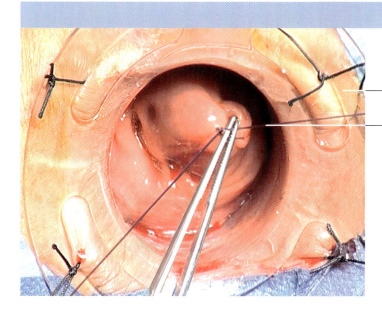

Tying the suture loosely

Circular Anal Dilator

First parachute suture

Nodal point 3 — Placing additional parachute sutures

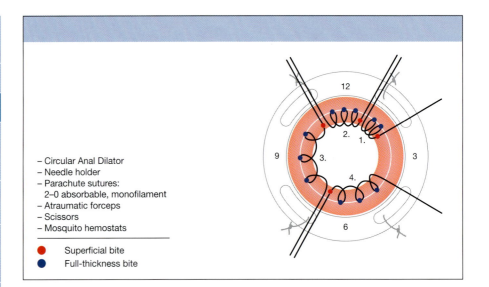

– Circular Anal Dilator
– Needle holder
– Parachute sutures:
  2–0 absorbable, monofilament
– Atraumatic forceps
– Scissors
– Mosquito hemostats

● Superficial bite
● Full-thickness bite

Place the first bite of the second parachute suture superficially on top of the prolapse at around 1 o'clock and not more than 1 cm away from the first parachute suture.

Position the following three to four full-thickness bites as a running suture counterclockwise from 1 to 11 o'clock, capturing the apex of the prolapse. Perform these bites deep enough to expose the prolapse and to gain solid traction on it. With the second parachute suture, capture 2–3 cm of the tissue circumferentially.

Tie the suture loosely in order to allow for good traction on the captured tissue.

> **Make sure to place the full-thickness bites of the parachute suture deep enough to expose the prolapse, and tie the suture loosely to gain good traction on the captured tissue (→ p. 53, III-2)!**

Connect the ends of the threads with a Mosquito hemostat and keep the suture under traction.

Likewise, apply two to three additional parachute sutures counterclockwise from 11 to 4 o'clock by avoiding gaps larger than 1 cm between the individual parachute sutures.

The number of bites per suture and the number of parachute sutures may vary from case to case. Make sure to place enough parachute sutures to achieve symmetrical traction on the prolapse throughout the circumference, but be careful not to position too many sutures to avoid narrowing the rectal lumen and therefore complicating the introduction of the Contour® Transtar™ Curved Cutter Stapler later.

> **Make sure not to leave too much space between the individual parachute sutures and to place enough parachute sutures to achieve uniform traction on the prolapse without narrowing the rectal lumen (→ p. 55, III-7a)!**

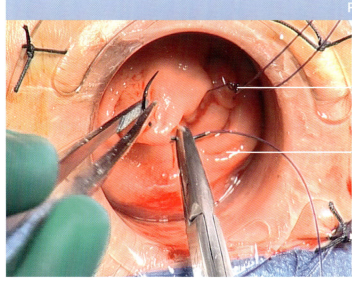

Placing the superficial bite of the second parachute suture

First parachute suture

Rectal prolapse

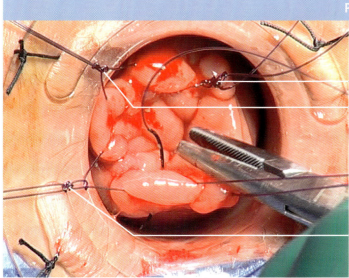

Placing a full-thickness bite of the fourth parachute suture

First parachute suture

Second parachute suture

Third parachute suture

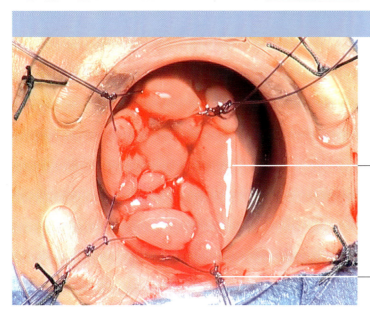

Parachute sutures under traction

Rectal prolapse

Fourth parachute suture

Nodal point 4   Placing a traction suture and introducing the Contour® Transtar™ Curved Cutter Stapler

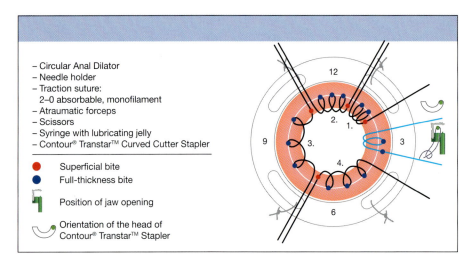

– Circular Anal Dilator
– Needle holder
– Traction suture:
  2–0 absorbable, monofilament
– Atraumatic forceps
– Scissors
– Syringe with lubricating jelly
– Contour® Transtar™ Curved Cutter Stapler

🔴 Superficial bite

🔵 Full-thickness bite

Position of jaw opening

Orientation of the head of Contour® Transtar™ Stapler

Place a traction suture at 3 o'clock at the base of the prolapse in the depth desired for its resection. Tie the suture tightly in order to reduce the prolapse thickness.

Make sure to tie the traction suture tightly in order to reduce the thickness of the prolapse!

Create a loop with the two ends of the thread.

Check that the cartridge is seated correctly in the jaws of the device.

Pay attention that the cartridge is seated correctly in the jaws of the Contour® Transtar™ Curved Cutter Stapler! Otherwise the gun might not fire or the retaining pin may not retract and may remain advanced through the tissue in the jaws of the instrument (→ p. 54, III-5)!

Lubricate the head of the Contour® Transtar™ Curved Cutter Stapler.

Apply traction to the parachute sutures, pulling the uppermost two sutures (first and second) upward and the lowermost sutures downward.

Hold the loop of the traction suture in the left hand. With the jaw opening facing the 3 o'clock position, pass the head of the Contour® Transtar™ Stapler through the loop from the right-hand side. Then pass the upper thread of the traction suture through the jaw opening so that it lies between the cartridge anvil and the cartridge module.

Now advance the head of the Contour® Transtar™ Stapler down the suture so that it lies well inside the rectal lumen. Ensure that it is completely surrounded by the rectal tissue captured by the parachute sutures in order not to close the rectum.

Pay attention to position the head of the device well inside the rectal lumen and to completely surround it by the captured tissue in order not to close the rectum (→ p. 55, III-7a)!

Position the head of the Contour® Transtar™ Stapler on the radial axis of the Circular Anal Dilator in order to longitudinally open the prolapse with the first cut.

First parachute suture

Traction suture

Fourth parachute suture

Inserting the Contour® Transtar™ Stapler into the traction suture loop

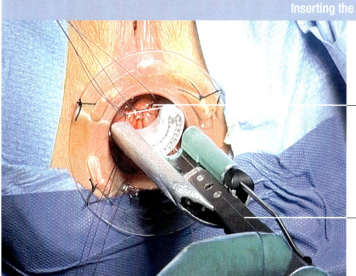

Uppermost parachute sutures

Traction suture loop

Placing the head of the Contour® Transtar™ Stapler on the radial axis of the Circular Anal Dilator

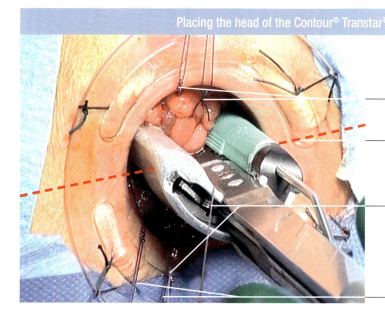

Uppermost parachute sutures

Radial axis

Traction suture loop

Lowermost parachute sutures

Nodal point 5 — Opening the rectal prolapse longitudinally

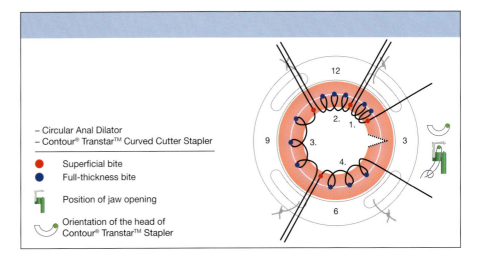

– Circular Anal Dilator
– Contour® Transtar™ Curved Cutter Stapler

● Superficial bite
● Full-thickness bite

Position of jaw opening

Orientation of the head of Contour® Transtar™ Stapler

Check visually that not too much tissue is captured in the jaws of the Contour® Transtar™ Stapler in order to enable firing and to achieve proper staple formation.

Make sure that not too much tissue is captured in the jaws of the device in order to enable firing and to achieve proper staple formation (→ p. 54, III-4; III-5)!

Close the retaining pin manually while still applying traction to the parachute sutures, so that the pin penetrates through the prolapse tissue and anchors the head of the Contour® Transtar™ Stapler.

In women, insert a finger into the vagina to ensure that it is not enclosed in the stapler.

Close the jaws of the device by squeezing the closure trigger and handle together. In women, re-check the vagina to ensure that the posterior vaginal wall is free from the rectal wall and the vaginal wall slides easily over the stapler.

It is mandatory to check that the vagina is mobile after closing the retaining pin and the stapler in order to avoid its incorporation in the staple line (→ p. 55, III-7b)!

In case of an incorporation of the vagina into the jaws of the device, re-open the Contour® Transtar™ Stapler, reposition the jaws, and close the retaining pin and the jaws again as described above.

To promote hemostasis, it is recommended to wait approximately 15 seconds after completely closing the instrument before firing.

It is recommended to wait approximately 15 seconds after completely closing the instrument before firing in order to promote hemostasis!

Fire the Contour® Transtar™ Stapler by squeezing the firing trigger.

Open the jaws of the instrument by pressing the release button and retract the retaining pin.

Remove the instrument carefully from the patient.

Inspect the staple line for proper staple formation, integrity and hemostasis (→ p. 54, III-4; III-6).

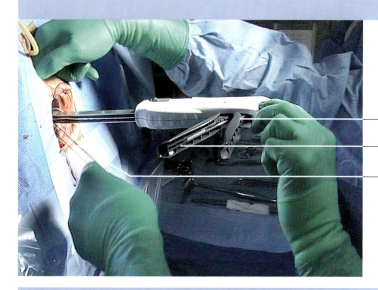

Closure trigger

Firing trigger

Parachute sutures

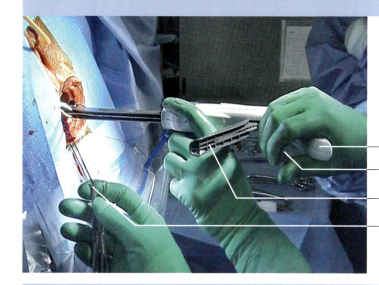

Handle

Closure trigger

Firing trigger

Parachute sutures

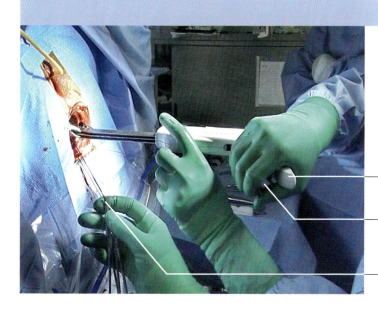

Handle

Firing trigger

Parachute sutures

Nodal point 6   Placing a marking suture and introducing the Contour® Transtar™ Curved Cutter Stapler

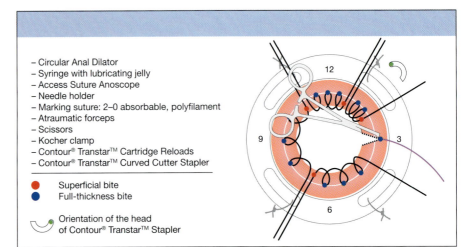

- Circular Anal Dilator
- Syringe with lubricating jelly
- Access Suture Anoscope
- Needle holder
- Marking suture: 2–0 absorbable, polyfilament
- Atraumatic forceps
- Scissors
- Kocher clamp
- Contour® Transtar™ Cartridge Reloads
- Contour® Transtar™ Curved Cutter Stapler

🔴 Superficial bite
🔵 Full-thickness bite

Orientation of the head of Contour® Transtar™ Stapler

Lubricate the Access Suture Anoscope, then introduce it. Place a marking suture at the apex of the opened prolapse to mark the ending of the following circumferential resection. Remove the anoscope.

Position a Kocher clamp parallel to the upper staple line and as close as possible to the apex of the opened prolapse in order to ensure the correct depth of the circumferential resection and to enable easy handling of the prolapse tissue.

> **Take care that the end part of the Kocher clamp is placed as close as possible to the apex of the opening line in order to resect the prolapse at the correct depth and to ensure proper seating of the device (→ p. 53, III-1; III-2; III-3)!**

Apply gentle and uniform traction to the parachute sutures. Then introduce the reloaded and lubricated Contour® Transtar™ Stapler with jaws opening facing the 3 o'clock position.

Rotate the instrument counterclockwise and gently pull the prolapse inside the jaws until the apex is seated in the deepest part. Pull the parachute sutures downward to the shaft of the Contour® Transtar™ Stapler while drawing the prolapse tissue into the jaws.

> **Make sure to pull the parachute sutures downward to the shaft of the device while drawing the prolapse tissue into the jaws (→ p. 53, III-1; III-2)!**

Make sure not to resect more than one quarter of the circumference per firing in order not to capture too much tissue in the jaws of the Contour® Transtar™ Stapler to avoid staple dehiscence or spiraling.

> **Pay attention not to go too fast along the circumference of the prolapse and not to capture too much tissue in the jaws of the Contour® Transtar™ Stapler to avoid staple dehiscence or spiraling (→ p. 53, III-1; III-2; p. 54, III-4)!**

Ensure that the head of the Contour® Transtar™ Stapler is positioned parallel to the Circular Anal Dilator.

> **Make sure to position the head of the device parallel to the Circular Anal Dilator!**

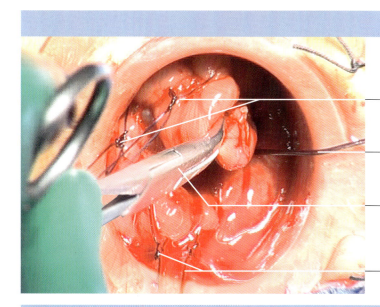

Marking suture

Needle holder

Positioning a Kocher clamp

First and second parachute suture

Marking suture

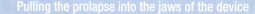

Kocher clamp

Third and fourth parachute suture

Pulling the prolapse into the jaws of the device

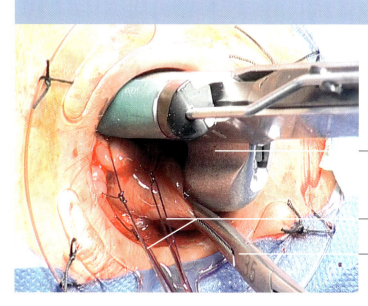

Head of Contour® Transtar™ Stapler

Parachute sutures

Kocher clamp

Nodal point 7 — Performing the first circumferential cut

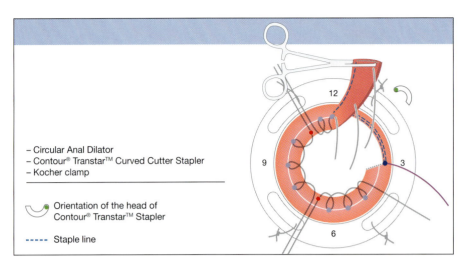

– Circular Anal Dilator
– Contour® Transtar™ Curved Cutter Stapler
– Kocher clamp

Orientation of the head of Contour® Transtar™ Stapler

- - - - Staple line

Check visually that not too much tissue is captured in the jaws of the Contour® Transtar™ Stapler in order to enable firing and to achieve proper staple formation.

Make sure that not too much tissue is captured in the jaws of the device in order to enable firing and to achieve proper staple formation (→ p. 54, III-4; III-5)!

Close the retaining pin manually while still applying traction to the parachute sutures, so that the pin penetrates through the prolapse tissue and anchors the head of the Contour® Transtar™ Stapler.

In women, insert a finger into the vagina to ensure that it is not enclosed in the stapler.

Close the jaws of the device by squeezing the closure trigger and handle together. In women, re-check the vagina to ensure that the posterior vaginal wall is free from the rectal wall and the vaginal wall slides easily over the stapler.

It is mandatory to check that the vagina is mobile after closing the retaining pin and the stapler to avoid its incorporation in the staple line (→ p. 55, III-7b)!

In case of an incorporation of the vagina into the jaws of the device, re-open the Contour® Transtar™ Stapler, reposition the jaws, and close the retaining pin and the jaws again as described above.

To promote hemostasis, it is recommended to wait approximately 15 seconds after completely closing the instrument before firing.

It is recommended to wait approximately 15 seconds after completely closing the instrument before firing in order to promote hemostasis!

Fire the Contour® Transtar™ Stapler by squeezing the firing trigger.

Open the jaws of the instrument by pressing the release button and retract the retaining pin.

Remove the instrument carefully from the patient.

Inspect the staple line for proper staple formation, integrity and hemostasis (→ p. 54, III-4; III-6).

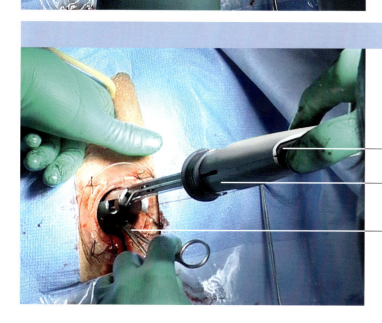

Contour® Transtar™ Stapler

Retaining pin actuator

Pushing the release button after firing

Release button

Contour® Transtar™ Stapler

Kocher clamp

47

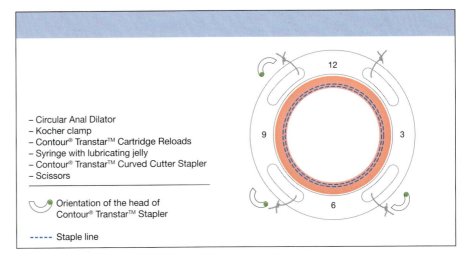

– Circular Anal Dilator
– Kocher clamp
– Contour® Transtar™ Cartridge Reloads
– Syringe with lubricating jelly
– Contour® Transtar™ Curved Cutter Stapler
– Scissors

⌣● Orientation of the head of Contour® Transtar™ Stapler

----- Staple line

Continue with the resection along the circumference as described in nodal points 6 and 7. Start with the introduction of the reloaded and lubricated Contour® Transtar™ Stapler and apply gentle and uniform traction to the parachute sutures throughout the procedure to achieve regular and proper circumferential resection.

It is mandatory to apply uniform traction to the parachute sutures throughout the procedure in order to ensure that a consistent amount of tissue is resected all along the circumference (→ p. 53, III-1; III-2; III-3)!

For the remaining circumferential resection, perform three or more cuts. The number of firings may vary from case to case. Digitally examine the rectal lumen between individual firings in order to avoid (partially) closing the rectum.

It is important to digitally examine the rectal lumen after each firing in order to avoid (partially) closing the rectum (→ p. 55, III-7a)!

The third and subsequent firings are the most difficult because there is a higher risk of resecting too superficially or too deeply. To avoid spiraling-in, spiraling-out or dog ears, complete each resection at the same distance from the anal verge as the starting point.

Ensure that all resections are completed at the same distance from the anal verge as the starting point and not more distal or proximal in order to avoid spiraling-in, spiraling-out or dog ears (→ p. 53, III-1; III-2; III-3)!

With the last firing, be sure to cut the remaining prolapse tissue completely and at the same depth as the marking suture. To this end, capture the entire remaining tissue in the jaws of the Contour® Transtar™ Stapler and close the retaining pin under vision freely and not through the tissue.

With the last firing, take care to cut the remaining prolapse tissue completely and at the correct depth in order to avoid spiraling-in, spiraling-out or dog ears (→ p. 53, III-1; III-2; III-3)!

After the last firing, remove the resected prolapse along with the Kocher clamp and cut the marking suture with scissors.

Inspect the staple line for proper staple formation, integrity and hemostasis (→ p. 54, III-4; III-6).

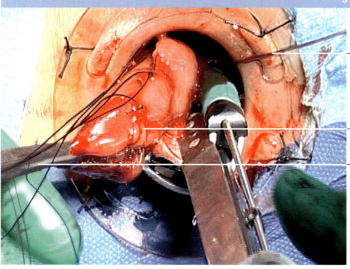

Placing the head of the Contour® Transtar™ Stapler

Kocher clamp

Rectal prolapse

Marking suture

Pulling the remaining prolapse tissue into the jaws of the device

Marking suture

Rectal prolapse

Kocher clamp

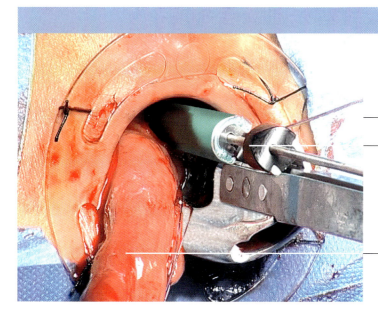

Placing the head of the device for the last cut

Marking suture

Head of Contour® Transtar™ Stapler

Rectal prolapse

Nodal point 9 — Finishing the operation

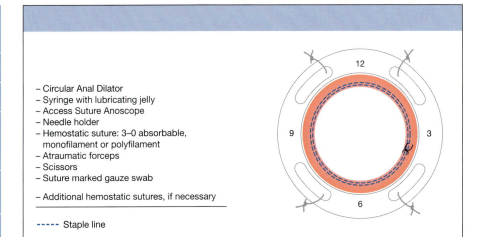

– Circular Anal Dilator
– Syringe with lubricating jelly
– Access Suture Anoscope
– Needle holder
– Hemostatic suture: 3–0 absorbable, monofilament or polyfilament
– Atraumatic forceps
– Scissors
– Suture marked gauze swab

– Additional hemostatic sutures, if necessary

----- Staple line

At the end of the procedure, examine the staple line carefully using the lubricated Access Suture Anoscope. Check particularly for proper staple formation and hemostasis (→ p. 54, III-4; III-6).

Reinforce the 3 o'clock end of the staple line with a suture regardless of the need for hemostasis or closure of defects.

It is important to place a suture at the end of the staple line in order to reinforce the anastomosis!

In case of bleeding, or where fat tissue or another suspicious zone is visible, place additional hemostatic sutures on the staple line in order to prevent bleeding or an incomplete anastomosis.

Make sure to place additional hemostatic sutures on fat tissue and suspicious zones in the staple line in order to avoid bleeding or an incomplete anastomosis (→ p. 54, III-4; III-6)!

Remove the Access Suture Anoscope carefully.

Insert a suture marked gauze swab transanally with its distal part visible from the outside to detect postoperative rectal bleeding.

Remove the fixation sutures and the Circular Anal Dilator.

Perform a vaginal examination with a speculum.

Take out the transurethral catheter.

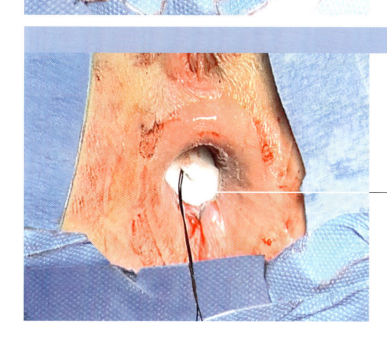

Hemostatic suture

Circular Anal Dilator

Inlying suture marked gauze swab

Suture marked gauze swab

Management of difficult situations, complications and mistakes

Spiraling-in 1

Spiraling-in can occur especially when the 3rd and the following circumferential cut does not end at the same depth as the prevoius circumferential cuts (starting at 3 o'clock) but proximal to it. This can lead to leaving an island of tissue between the two staple lines with a possible risk of ischemia.

To avoid spiraling-in, make sure that with every firing the same amount of prolapse is resected. With the last firing make sure that the final resection is at the level of the marking suture. Possibly include the marking suture in the last firing, and make sure that the retaining pin is closed under vision, freely and not through the prolapse tissue.

If spiraling-in has occurred, check for defects and isolated islands of mucosa (which could be exposed to ischemia), and reinforce them with running sutures.

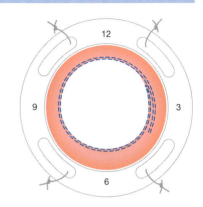

Spiraling-out 2

Spiraling-out can occur when the parachute sutures are not all placed at a uniform, correct depth around the circumference. It also can happen if the device is rotated too much and is not properly fed with the prolapse. This can lead to a high suture line and therefore to the resection of an incomplete specimen.

To avoid spiraling-out, ensure that the full-thickness bites of the parachute sutures are positioned deep enough to capture the whole prolapse that needs to be resected and to resect a maximum of one quarter of the circumference per firing. Take care to perform the third and subsequent firings very carefully to avoid resecting the prolapse too superficially.

In case spiraling-out occurs, start again at the correct level part way around, replacing the parachute sutures and excising the badly positioned portion of the staple line.

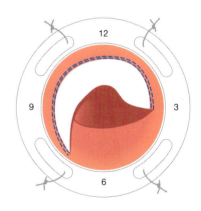

Dog ears 3

Dogs ears can occur when the head of the Contour® Transtar™ Stapler is not pushed down to the apex of the previous cut.

To avoid dogs ears, make sure each resection is completed at the same level of the previous circumferential cut.

In the event of a dog ear, stitch over the dog ear to reduce its size. If the dog ear is too large, use one more cartridge to resect it.

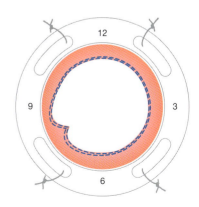

4 Vulnerable areas in staple line

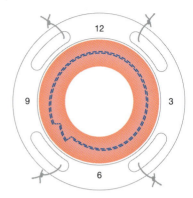

When using the Contour® Transtar™ Stapler, it is important to understand that the knife cuts between two lines of staples on the outer curve and only one line of staples on the inner side. Vulnerable areas of single staple line can be left inside the patient if the head of the Contour® Transtar™ Stapler is not placed deeply enough during the third and subsequent firings.

To avoid areas of single staple line it is important to place the head of the Contour® Transtar™ Stapler during the third and subsequent firings as deeply as during the second cut to perform a continuous staple line.

Inspect the staple line carefully after each firing and at the end of the procedure.

In case of vulnerable areas, small remaining defects between the staples, or suspicion of weak areas in the staple line, reinforce it with additional sutures during or at the end of the procedure.

5 Incorrect closing of the retaining pin

The retaining pin consists of two parts: one in the instrument and one in the cartridge. The pin in the instrument advances the pin in the cartridge when the device is closed. Therefore, if the cartridge is not seated properly or if too much tissue is captured in the jaws of the device, the gun might not fire or the retaining pin may not retract after firing and may remain advanced through the tissue in the jaws of the instrument.

If the retaining pin remains advanced through the tissue in the jaws of the device, retract it manually using a Kocher clamp.

6 Blood vessel injuries

a) Intraoperative bleeding

Examine the staple line carefully for proper hemostasis after each firing and at the end of the procedure.

In case of intraoperative bleeding, place hemostatic sutures on the staple line during or at the end of the procedure.

b) Postoperative bleeding

Check postoperatively for any rectal bleeding by leaving a suture marked gauze swab in the rectum after the procedure.

In case of postoperative bleeding, place hemostatic sutures on the staple line.

a) Rectum

Narrowing of the rectum can occur due to the positioning of too many parachute sutures. This can complicate the introduction of the Contour® Transtar™ Stapler into the rectum.

To avoid this, place enough sutures to achieve a symmetrical traction on the prolapse throughout the circumference, but be careful not to place too many sutures.

In case of a narrowed rectum, replace the parachute sutures.

Complete or partial closing of the rectum can occur if tissue from the opposite rectal wall is inadvertently caught while the parachute sutures are being placed, due to improper positioning of the head of the Contour® Transtar™ Stapler inside the rectal lumen, or during incorrect circumferential stapling.

To avoid closing the rectum, use the Access Suture Anoscope or a mounted gauze swab to place the parachute sutures and position the head of the Contour® Transtar™ Stapler well inside the rectal lumen before firing. Between the individual firings, check regularly where the rectal lumen is by careful digital examination.

If the rectum is accidentally closed, it is necessary to identify the suture line closing the lumen, to open it fully, and to close the rectal wall defects with running sutures. A protective stoma is mandatory, if correction of the rectal wall defects is not satisfactory.

b) Vagina in women

Injury to or closing of the vagina can occur when tissue from the wall opposing the rectum is inadvertently caught while the parachute sutures are being placed, during closure of the retaining pin, and during circumferential stapling when vaginal tissue is incorporated in the staple line.

To avoid any injury to the vagina use the Access Suture Anoscope or a mounted gauze swab to place the parachute sutures and perform the first longitudinal firing at 3 o'clock. Carefully check that the vagina is mobile after closing of the retaining pin and the stapler before every firing.

If the vagina is trapped in the jaws of the device during firing, a communication (fistula) between the rectum and the vagina will be created. In such a situation, the vagina and the rectum should be separated with smooth dissection around the communication created. The staples around the defect should be removed. The defect in the vagina is then closed with absorbable sutures. Depending on the size of the recto-vaginal fistula a protective stoma may be fashioned in order to allow the healing of the defect.

c) Anal sphincter

Injury to the anal sphincter can occur if it is dilated too excessively with the Obturator at the beginning of the operation. This can lead to anal incontinence.

To avoid any injury to the anal sphincter do not dilate it too excessively with the Obturator.

What is Obstructed Defecation Syndrome (ODS)?

1.   Key points
2.   Definition and symptoms
3.   Main etiologies
3.1   Functional
3.2   Mechanical
3.2.1   Low rectal redundancy
3.2.2   Complex pelvic prolapses

Patient selection for STARR

1.   Rationale for selection of patients to undergo STARR procedure
2.   Patient inclusion criteria – symptoms of ODS
3.   Patient selection after dynamic imaging with special reference to the STARR procedure
3.1   ODS Scores
3.2   Defecography and MRI
4.   Patient exclusion criteria for the STARR procedure

Postoperative management

1.   Analgesia
2.   Wound care
3.   Mobilization
4.   Nutrition
5.   Discharge

Sample operation note

Bibliography

List of key words

What is Obstructed Defecation Syndrome (ODS)?

1. Key points

Obstructed Defecation Syndrome (ODS) is secondary to various etiologies, including rectal stasis disorders.

Internal rectal prolapse and rectocele are frequent in patients with ODS.

Low rectal redundancy is the anatomical common feature for patients with these defects, meaning that rectocele and intussusception are different dynamic aspects of the same rectal deformity.

STARR corrects low rectal redundancy, thus aiming to improve ODS symptoms and quality of life in selected patients.

2. Definition and symptoms

Classically, ODS is defined by symptoms evoking the inability to satisfactorily evacuate the rectum in the presence of a desire to defecate.

Symptoms of ODS are rarely clearly expressed by patients. One of the most common complaints is: "Doctor, I have hemorrhoids!"; rarely it is: "I suffer from constipation"; unfortunately, it is never: "Doctor, I have Obstructed Defecation Syndrome with rectocele and internal rectal prolapse." Therefore, symptoms of ODS should be specifically searched for. They may be:

• Extreme straining to defecate
• Pain on defecation
• Extended time on the toilet
• Perineal pain/discomfort when standing
• Feeling of incomplete evacuation
• False urgency
• Fragmented defecation
• Vaginal, perineal or rectal digitation
• Use of laxatives or enemas

3. Main etiologies

These are classified as functional and mechanical.

3.1 Functional

• Slow-transit constipation explains symptoms of obstructed defecation mainly because of the difficulty of expelling hard and small stools. Furthermore, it is often associated with mechanical causes of ODS. It has even been suggested that in some patients slow colonic transit may be secondary to defecation disorders.

• Defective rectal motility and/or sensitivity, either primary (rectal inertia) or secondary to drugs.

• Pelvi-rectal dyssynergia secondary to either an absence of relaxation (or a paradoxical contraction) of striated musculature, or an inefficient relaxation of the internal anal sphincter (Hirschsprung disease, Chagas disease, ...). This condition may be associated with mechanical prolapses found in patients with ODS.

3.2 Mechanical

- Rectal redundancy is the most common condition explaining both internal rectal prolapse and rectocele formation. If isolated, this condition is therefore a good indication for STARR.

- Complex pelvic prolapses where rectal deformity is caused, or increased, by other organ prolapses such as enterocele, sigmoidocele, and urogenital prolapse. Descending perineum is rather the consequence of diffuse pelvi-perineal neuro-muscular alteration than a specific condition impeding rectal evacuation.

Paradoxically, these extrarectal deformities may help rectal emptying by the pressure they exert during straining efforts on the anterior wall of the rectum (enterocele, uterine prolapse) or its lengthening (descending perineum). The rectal prolapse is then "compensated" and ODS symptoms may be minor.

Clinical examination alone is not sensitive enough to evaluate these complex conditions; therefore, exhaustive radiological evaluation is necessary (defecography with multivisceral opacification, dynamic MRI) when the indication for surgery depends on anatomical defects.

3.2.1 Low rectal redundancy

Figures 1 and 2 clearly illustrate the fact that rectocele and internal rectal prolapse are both expressions of low rectal redundancy. Transanal low rectal resection will shorten and straighten the rectal wall, thus correcting rectocele and internal rectal prolapse.

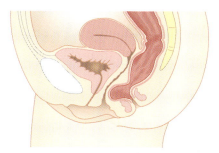 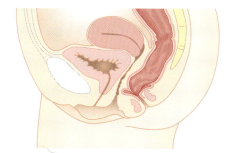

Fig. 1 Anterior rectocele   Fig. 2 Internal rectal prolapse

Two cases are illustrated, demonstrating the two main anatomical presentations of low rectal redundancy: anterior rectocele and internal rectal prolapse (figures 3–8). It is important to note that dynamic rectal alterations are best demonstrated at the end of the straining effort, when rectal emptying is maximal.

Case 1: Woman with an isolated recto-anal internal rectal prolapse

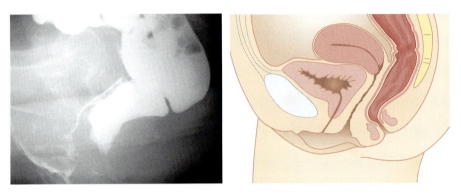

Fig. 3   Patient at rest during dynamic X-ray pelvic examination, compared with schematic representation.

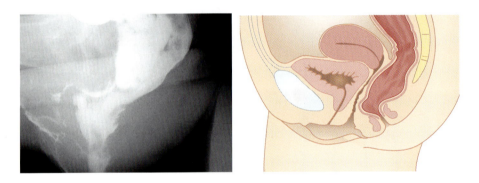

Fig. 4   Same patient during the first stage of rectal evacuation.

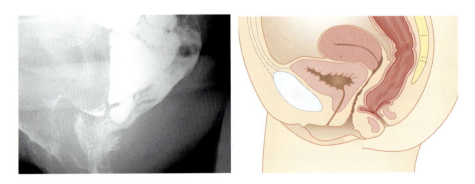

Fig. 5   Same patient during maximal straining effort. Following rectal evacuation recto-anal prolapse is clearly visualized.

Case 2: Woman with recto-anal internal rectal prolapse and rectocele

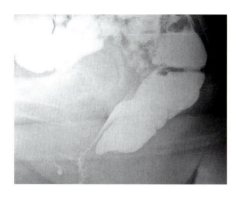 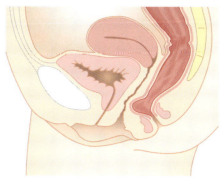

Fig. 6   Patient at rest during dynamic X-ray pelvic examination, compared with schematic representation.

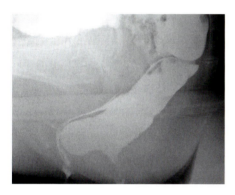 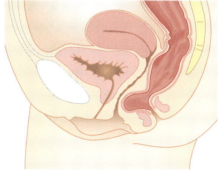

Fig. 7   Same patient during straining effort. Rectocele is bulging anteriorly towards vagina lumen, internal rectal prolapse is not apparent.

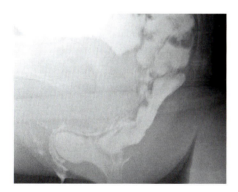 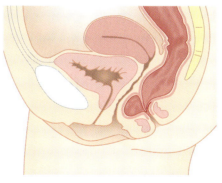

Fig. 8   Same patient during maximal straining effort following rectal evacuation. Rectocele evacuation is incomplete and recto-anal prolapse is demonstrated.

3.2.2 Complex pelvic prolapses

In these conditions, rectal deformity is associated with complex pelvic organ displacement (enterocele, sigmoidocele, vaginal vault, uterine or bladder prolapse). Case 3 illustrates the association of an internal rectal prolapse with an enterocele (figures 9–11).

Case 3: Woman with past history of hysterectomy, presenting an internal rectal prolapse associated with an enterocele

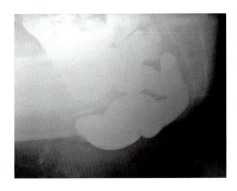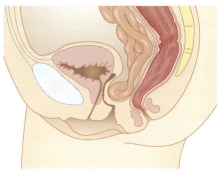

Fig. 9   Patient at rest.

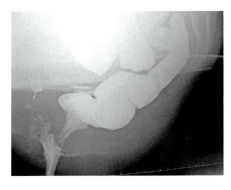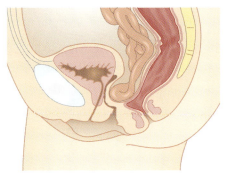

Fig. 10   Same patient during straining effort at first stage of rectal evacuation.

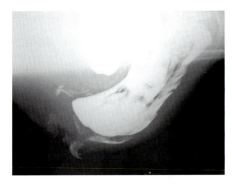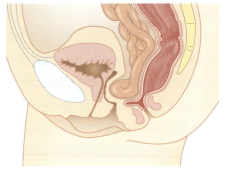

Fig. 11   Same patient during maximal straining effort at the end of rectal evacuation. An enterocele is protruding between vagina and rectum wall down to perineal plane.

1. Rationale for selection of patients to undergo STARR procedure

As it straightens and shortens the low rectal segment (figures 12 and 13), STARR aims to correct low rectal redundancy. When this condition is associated with ODS symptoms, STARR will correct anatomy thus suppressing ODS symptoms and therefore improving quality of life.

As explained in the following chapters, selection of patients is the key for an optimal balance between positive effects and potential morbidity.

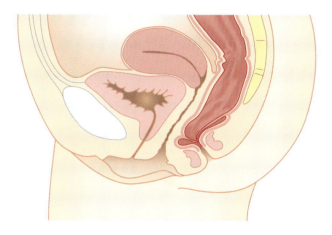

Before STARR

Fig. 12   Rectal deformation associated with low rectal redundancy.

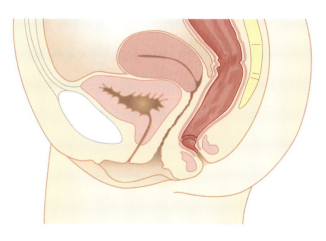

After STARR

Fig. 13   Correction of low rectal redundancy after transanal resection of lower rectal segment.

Patient inclusion criteria – symptoms of ODS

1 Evacuation by prolonged or repeated straining

2 Frequent calls to defecate prior to or following evacuation

3 Use of digital means to effect evacuation

4 Laxative and/or enema use required to defecate

5 Sense of incomplete evacuation

6 Excessive time spent on the toilet

7 Pelvic pressure, rectal discomfort, and perineal pain

2. Patient inclusion criteria – symptoms of ODS

Frequently, in patients with ODS, an internal rectal prolapse and/or rectocele is found during clinical examination. Patients with the combination of the above symptoms (→ p. 58) and these anatomical findings may be candidates for further assessment and possible surgical treatment.

As symptoms, morphological findings, and potential treatment options are wide-ranging in ODS patients, a careful diagnostic assessment is recommended. It is a prerequisite to exclude colorectal malignancy and inflammatory bowel disease by colonoscopy. Conservative treatment such as diet, stool regulation including enemas and laxatives, pelvic floor retraining, and biofeedback improves constipation symptoms in a considerable proportion of patients. Surgery (including the STARR procedure) may be considered in patients for whom conservative treatment options have failed and where there is an underlying morphological abnormality such as internal rectal prolapse and/or rectocele.

3. Patient selection after dynamic imaging with special reference to the STARR procedure

Patient selection is the key to successful therapy of ODS. Following diagnostic assessment, those patients who may be considered as suitable candidates for the STARR procedure should have failed prior conservative treatment.

To provide a standardized decision-making algorithm, treatment options after dynamic imaging were differentiated in relation to the most common clinical findings (internal rectal prolapse with or without rectocele) in patients suffering from ODS (see next page). If internal rectal prolapse and rectocele are confirmed clinically and morphologically, and diagnostic assessment can rule out significant combined pathologies, the STARR procedure can be recommended as first option. However, if internal rectal prolapse and rectocele are combined with other pelvic floor diseases, such as enterocele, sigmoidocele, or urogenital prolapse, a treatment of these associated disorders (as per local practice) should be recommended first. In experienced pelvic floor centers, treatment of enterocele can be combined with the STARR procedure. If clinically and morphologically confirmed internal rectal prolapse and rectocele are associated with pelvic dyssynergia, the primary treatment option should be conservative (e.g. biofeedback). If fecal incontinence is associated with internal rectal prolapse and rectocele, a tailored therapy with special reference to sphincter function should be initiated.

STARR Algorithm

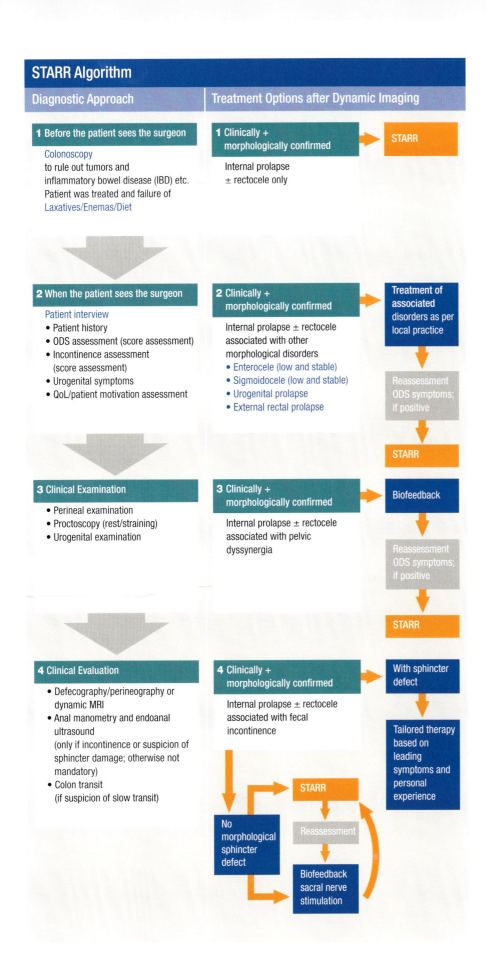

Diagnostic Approach

1 Before the patient sees the surgeon

Colonoscopy
to rule out tumors and
inflammatory bowel disease (IBD) etc.
Patient was treated and failure of
Laxatives/Enemas/Diet

2 When the patient sees the surgeon

Patient interview
• Patient history
• ODS assessment (score assessment)
• Incontinence assessment
  (score assessment)
• Urogenital symptoms
• QoL/patient motivation assessment

3 Clinical Examination

• Perineal examination
• Proctoscopy (rest/straining)
• Urogenital examination

4 Clinical Evaluation

• Defecography/perineography or
  dynamic MRI
• Anal manometry and endoanal
  ultrasound
  (only if incontinence or suspicion of
  sphincter damage; otherwise not
  mandatory)
• Colon transit
  (if suspicion of slow transit)

Treatment Options after Dynamic Imaging

**1 Clinically +
morphologically confirmed**

Internal prolapse
± rectocele only

→ STARR

**2 Clinically +
morphologically confirmed**

Internal prolapse ± rectocele
associated with other
morphological disorders
• Enterocele (low and stable)
• Sigmoidocele (low and stable)
• Urogenital prolapse
• External rectal prolapse

→ **Treatment of
associated**
disorders as per
local practice

↓

Reassessment
ODS symptoms;
if positive

↓

STARR

**3 Clinically +
morphologically confirmed**

Internal prolapse ± rectocele
associated with pelvic
dyssynergia

→ Biofeedback

↓

Reassessment
ODS symptoms;
if positive

↓

STARR

**4 Clinically +
morphologically confirmed**

Internal prolapse ± rectocele
associated with fecal
incontinence

→ **With sphincter
defect**

↓

Tailored therapy
based on
leading
symptoms and
personal
experience

No
morphological
sphincter
defect

STARR

Reassessment

Biofeedback
sacral nerve
stimulation

3.1 ODS Scores

A variety of ODS scores exist, some of which are validated and others are not. In general, scores are useful to quantify patient's symptoms; however, they cannot be used as decision criteria for surgery. The main use of these scores is in the assessment of patient's symptoms before and after surgery, and to facilitate comparisons between clinical studies and between different medical institutions.

Symptom Severity Score

1. Need for laxatives/enemas	0 1 2 3 4	6. Incomplete bowel opening	0 1 2 3 4
2. Unsuccessful attempts to open bowels	0 1 2 3 4	7. Bleeding on bowel opening	0 1 2 3 4
3. Low frequency of bowel movements	0 1 2 3 4	8. Incontinence/soiling	0 1 2 3 4
4. Increased time of straining to open bowels	0 1 2 3 4	9. Difficulty to withstand urge to open bowels	0 1 2 3 4
5. Pain on bowel opening	0 1 2 3 4	0 = none of the time 1 = a little of the time 2 = some of the time 3 = most of the time 4 = all of the time	

ODS Score (by Longo)

Defecation Frequency	Straining Intensity	Duration

0 = 1–2 defecations/1–2 days
1 = 2 defecations/week or
  3 defecations or attempts/day
2 = 1 defecation/week or
  4 defecations or attempts/day
3 = less than 1x/week or
  4 defecations or attempts/day
	0 = none to light
	1 = moderate
	2 = intensive
		1 = short time
		2 = prolonged or many times

Feeling of Incomplete Evacuation	**Rectoperineal Pain/Discomfort**	**Activity Reduction**
0 = never 1 = less than or 1x/week 2 = 2x/week 3 = more than 2x/week	0 = never 1 = less than or 1x/week 2 = 2x/week 3 = more than 2x/week	0 = never 1 = less than 25 % of activity 4 = 25–50 % of activity 6 = more than 50 % of activity
Laxatives	**Enemas**	**Digitation**
0 = never 1 = fewer than 25 % of defecations 3 = 25–50 % of defecations 5 = more than 50 % of defecations 7 = always	0 = never 1 = fewer than 25 % of defecations 3 = 25–50 % of defecations 5 = more than 50 % of defecations 7 = always	0 = never 1 = fewer than 25 % of defecations 3 = 25–50 % of defecations 5 = more than 50 % of defecations 7 = always

Incontinence Score (by Wexner)					
	Solid	Liquid	Gas	Required Pad	Lifestyle Alteration
Never	0	0	0	0	0
Rarely	1	1	1	1	1
Sometimes	2	2	2	2	2
Usually	3	3	3	3	3
Always	4	4	4	4	4

Never
Rarely: Less than once per month
Sometimes: Once or more than once per month, less than once per week
Usually: Once or more than once per week, less than once per day
Always: More than once per day

3.2 Defecography and MRI

Evacuatory proctography (defecography) is a method of dynamic assessment of defecation. It consists in the administration of a barium contrast in the rectum to evaluate the defecatory activity. Vaginal and intestinal contrast are also administered for a more complete pelvic evaluation. It provides an understanding of pelvic-floor physiopathology, but this must be interpreted cautiously because findings may correlate poorly with symptomatic assessment. Video recordings are obtained with the patient at rest, squeezing and straining without evacuation, and during evacuation of the rectal contrast (→ p. 60–62). Anorectal angle, pelvic floor descent, morphology of rectal wall and other pelvic pathologies (as sigmoidocele or enterocele) are evaluated with this method.

MRI is a noninvasive technique that does not require any special preparation. It has been shown to provide a more complete evaluation of the pelvic pathology, especially of the mucosal alterations and the anterior pelvic compartment when compared with evacuatory proctography.

4. Patient exclusion criteria for the STARR procedure

Precise exclusion criteria have been developed by the STARR Pioneers on the basis of technical aspects and with special reference to preventing septic complications.

Patient exclusion criteria

1 Active anorectal infection
2 Concurrent severe anorectal pathology
3 Proctitis (induced by IBD, radiation)
4 Enterocele at rest (low, stable)
5 Chronic diarrhea

Relative patient exclusion criteria

1 Presence of foreign material adjacent to the rectum (i.e. mesh)
2 Previous transanal surgery (i.e. rectal anastomosis)
3 Concurrent psychiatric disorder

Postoperative management

1. Analgesia

Prescription of simple analgesia (e.g. paracetamol/acetaminophen) is sufficient in most cases.

Avoid opioids if possible because of their constipating side effects.

2. Wound care

Because the staple line is endorectal no special wound care is indicated.

Pads should be given to protect underwear from soiling. Advise the patient that mucus and a small amount of blood are not uncommon in the first 5–7 days.

Measure the patients' body temperature daily in order to detect an occult infection early.

3. Mobilization

Depending on anesthetic after effects and circulatory stability, mobilize the patient as soon as possible postoperatively.

4. Nutrition

As soon as the effect of the anesthesia is gone allow the patient to eat and drink.

Prescribe the patient a stool softener for the first 3–4 postoperative weeks.

5. Discharge

Discharge the patient on the second or third day. Prior to discharge make sure that the patient is mobilized, has passed urine, is pain free, and is tolerating a normal diet.

Date:	Operating surgeon:
Patient's name:	Assistant:
Indication: Defecation disorder with a low rectal prolapse	Scrub nurse: Anesthetist:
Operation: Stapled Transanal Rectal Resection (STARR) with Contour® Transtar™ Curved Cutter Stapler Procedure Set	

Patient under general anesthesia, placed in lithotomy and 30° Trendelenburg position.

Four perianal sutures are placed at 1, 11, 7 and 5 o'clock. The Obturator is inserted and the anal sphincter is dilated. The Circular Anal Dilator and the Obturator are inserted and the Circular Anal Dilator is fixed to the anal margin with the four perianal sutures.

The prolapse is exposed through the dilator with a mounted gauze swab. The Access Suture Anoscope is inserted with the open window positioned at 2 o'clock. The superficial bite of the first parachute suture is placed at 2 o'clock. Then the anoscope is removed. Three full-thickness bites are positioned as a running suture counterclockwise from 2 to 1 o'clock, capturing the apex of the prolapse. The suture is tied loosely. The ends of the threads are connected with a Mosquito hemostat and kept under traction. Likewise, three additional parachute sutures are placed counterclockwise from 1 to 4 o'clock.

A traction suture is placed over full prolapse height at 3 o'clock and is tied tightly. With the ends of the threads a loop is created. While traction is applied to the parachute sutures, the head of the Contour® Transtar™ Curved Cutter Stapler is inserted into the loop of the traction suture. The head is positioned well inside the rectal lumen on the radial axis of the dilator. The retaining pin and the jaws of the device are closed. The mobility of the vagina is checked manually; it is not enclosed in the stapler. The prolapse is longitudinally opened at 3 o'clock.

The anoscope is introduced and a marking suture is placed at the apex of the opened prolapse. After the anoscope is removed, a Kocher clamp is positioned parallel to the upper staple line of the opened prolapse. While traction is applied to the parachute sutures, the reloaded stapler is introduced into the anal canal with the jaw opening facing 3 o'clock. The prolapse is pulled into the jaws, while the device is rotated counterclockwise. The head of the stapler is positioned parallel to the dilator. The retaining pin and the jaws of the device are closed, the vagina is checked and is not enclosed in the stapler. The stapler is fired and approximately the first quarter of the prolapse is resected. The staple line is inspected. There is no dehiscence or bleeding visible.

Three successive applications allow complete circumferential resection of the prolapse. Before each firing the mobility of the vagina is checked manually. Following the last cut the Kocher clamp is removed. At the end of the procedure the anoscope is introduced and the staple line is checked. The suture line is regular without dehiscence. The 3 o'clock end of the staple line is reinforced with a suture. Hemostatic sutures are performed, where necessary. Rectal prolapse is reduced.

Following removal of the anoscope, the height of the staple line is estimated to be at 6 cm from the anal margin. Five cartridges have been used. A suture marked gauze swab is introduced transanally. The fixation sutures and the dilator are removed.

The specimen is one piece. It is opened and demonstrates full-thickness rectal wall extirpation surrounded by rectal fat. Specimen size is 12 x 6 cm.

Bibliography

Altomare D.F., Spazzafumo L., Rinaldi M., Dodi G., Ghiselli R. & Piloni V. (2008). Set-up and statistical validation of a new scoring system for obstructed defaecation syndrome. *Colorectal Disease*, 10: 84-88.

Banister J.J., Davidson P., Timms J.M., Gibbons C. & Read N.W. (1987). Effect of stool size and consistency on defecation. *Gut*, 28: 1246-1250.

Boccasanta P., Venturi M., Stuto A., Bottini C., Caviglia A., Carriero A., Mascagni D., Mauri R., Sofo L. & Landolfi V. (2004). Stapled transanal rectal resection for outlet obstruction: A prospective, multicenter trial. *Diseases of the Colon & Rectum*, 47: 1285-1297.

Bremer S., Mellgren A., Holmström B. & Uden R. (1997). Pelvic anatomy and pathology is influenced by distention of the rectum. *Diseases of the Colon & Rectum*, 40: 1477-1483.

Carpenter W.B. (1874). *Principles of Mental Physiology: With their Applications to the Training and Discipline of the Mind and the Study of its Comorbid Conditions.* London: Henry S. King & Co.

Corman M.L., Carriero A., Hager T., Herold A., Jayne D.G., Lehur P.-A., Lomanto D., Longo A., Mellgren A.F., Nicholls J., Nystrom P.-O., Senagore A.J., Stuto A. & Wexner S.D. (2006). Consensus conference on the stapled transanal rectal resection (STARR) for disordered defecation. *Colorectal Disease*, 8: 98-101.

Dodi G., Pietroletti R., Milito G., Binda G. & Pescatori M. (2003). Bleeding, incontinence, pain and constipation after STARR transanal double stapling rectotomy for obstructed defecation. *Techniques in Coloproctology*, 7: 148-153.

Drossman D.A., Thompson G.W., Talley N.J., Funch-Jensen P., Janssens J. & Whitehead W.E. (1990). Identification of sub-groups of functional gastrointestinal disorders. *Gastroenterology International*, 3: 159-172.

Dvorkin L.S., Hetzer F., Scott S.M., Williams N.S., Gedroyc W. & Lunniss P.J. (2004). Open magnet MR defecography compared with evacuation proctography in the diagnosis and management of patients with rectal intussusception. *Colorectal Disease*, 1: 45-53.

Feltz D.L. & Landers D.M. (1983). The effects of mental practice on motor skill learning and performance: A meta-analysis. *Journal of Sport Psychology*, 5: 25-57.

Fucini C., Ronchi O. & Elbetti C. (2001). Electromyography of the pelvic floor musculature in the assessment of Obstructed Defecation Syndrome. *Diseases of the Colon & Rectum*, 44: 1168-1175.

Bibliography

Güler A.K., Immenroth M., Berg T., Bürger T. & Gawad K.A. (2006). Evaluation einer neu konzipierten Operationsfibel durch den Vergleich mit einer klassischen Operationslehre. *Posterpräsentation auf dem 123. Kongress der Deutschen Gesellschaft für Chirurgie vom 02.–05. Mai 2006 in Berlin.*

Halligan S., Thomas J. & Bartram C. (1995). Intrarectal pressures and balloon expulsion related to evacuation proctography. *Gut,* 37: 100-104.

Healy J.C., Halligan S., Reznek R.H., Watson S., Bartram C.l., Phillips R. & Amstrong P. (1997). Dynamic MR imaging compared with evacuation proctography when evaluating anorectal configuration and pelvic floor movement. *American Journal of Roentgenology,* 169: 775-779.

Immenroth M. (2003). *Mentales Training in der Medizin. Anwendung in der Chirurgie und Zahnmedizin.* Hamburg: Kovaç.

Immenroth M., Bürger T., Brenner J., Kemmler R., Nagelschmidt R., Eberspächer H. & Troidl H. (2005). Mentales Training in der Chirurgie. *Der Chirurg* BDC, 44: 21-25.

Immenroth M., Bürger T., Brenner J., Nagelschmidt R., Eberspächer H. & Troidl H. (2007). Mental Training in surgical education: A randomized controlled trial. *Annals of Surgery,* 245: 385-391.

Immenroth M., Eberspächer H. & Hermann H.D. (2008). Training kognitiver Fertigkeiten. In J. Beckmann & M. Kellmann (Hrsg.), *Enzyklopädie der Psychologie (D, V, 2) Anwendungen der Sportpsychologie* (119-176). Göttingen: Hogrefe.

Immenroth M., Eberspächer H., Nagelschmidt M., Troidl H., Bürger T., Brenner J., Berg T., Müller M. & Kemmler R. (2005). Mentales Training in der Chirurgie – Sicherheit durch ein besseres Training. Design und erste Ergebnisse einer Studie. *MIC,* 14: 69-74.

Jayne D. & Finan P.J. (2005). Stapled transanal rectal resection for obstructed defaecation and evidence-based practice. *British Journal of Surgery,* 92: 793-794.

Jayne D. & Stuto A. (2009). *Transanal Stapling Techniques for Anorectal Prolapse.* London: Springer.

Kaarlbom U., Pählman L., Nilsson S. & Graf W. (1995). Relationship between defecographic findings, rectal emptying, and colonic transit time in constipated patients. *Gut,* 36: 907-912.

Kiff E.S., Barnes P.R.H. & Swash M. (1984). Evidence of pudendal neuropathy in patients with perineal descent and chronic straining at stool. *Gut,* 25: 1279-1282.

Bibliography

Knowles C.H., Eccersley A.J., Scott S.M., Walker S.M., Reeves B. & Lunniss P.J. (2000). Linear discriminant analysis of symptoms in patients with chronic constipation: validation of a new scoring system (KESS). *Diseases of the Colon & Rectum*, 43: 1419-1426.

Koch A., Voderholzer W.A., Klauser A.G. & Müller-Lissner S. (1997). Symptoms in chronic constipation. *Diseases of the Colon & Rectum*, 40: 902-906.

Lenisa L., Schwandner O., Stuto A., Jayne D., Pigot F., Tuech J.J., Scherer R., Nugent K., Corbisier F., Espin Basany E. & Hetzer F. (in press). STARR with Contour® Transtar™ Stapler: Prospective Multicentre European Study. *Colorectal Disease*.

Longo A. (2003). Obstructed defecation because of rectal pathologies. Novel surgical treatment: Stapled transanal rectal resection (STARR). *Proceedings of the 14th Annual International Colorectal Disease Symposium, February 13-15, 2003 in Ft. Lauderdale, Florida*.

Lotze R.H. (1852). *Medicinische Psychologie und Physiologie der Seele*. Leipzig: Weidmann'sche Buchhandlung.

Mathur P., Ng K.-H. & Seow-Choen F. (2004). Stapled mucosectomy for rectocele repair: A preliminary report. *Diseases of the Colon & Rectum*, 47: 1978-1981.

Miller G.A. (1956). The magical number seven plus or minus two: Some limits on our capacity for processing information. *Psychological Review*, 63: 81-97.

Oliveira L., Pfeiffer J. & Wexner S.D. (1996). Physiology and clinical outcome of anterior sphincteroplasty. *British Journal of Surgery*, 83: 502-505.

Petersen S., Hellmich G., Schuster A., Lehmann D., Albert W. & Ludwig K. (2006). Stapled transanal rectal resection under laparoscopic surveillance for rectocele and concomitant enterocele. *Diseases of the Colon & Rectum*, 49: 1-5.

Pigot F., Castinel A., Juguet F., Marrel A., Deroche C. & Marquis P. (2001). Quality of life, symptoms of dyschezia, and anatomy after correction of rectal motility disorder. *Gastroentérologie Clinique et Biologique*, 25: 154-160.

Renzi A., Izzo D., Di Sarno G., Izzo G. & Di Martino N. (2006). Stapled transanal rectal resection to treat obstructed defecation caused by rectal intussusception and rectocele. *International Journal of Colorectal Disease*, 21: 661-667.

Schouten W.R., Gosselink M.J., Boerma M.O. & Ginai A.Z. (1998). Rectal wall contractility in response to an evoked urge to defecate in patients with obstructed defecation. *Diseases of the Colon & Rectum*, 41: 473-479.

Schwandner O., Stuto A., Jayne D., Lenisa L., Pigot F., Tuech J.J., Scherer R., Nugent K., Corbisier F., Espin Basany E. & Hetzer F. (2008). Decision-making algorithm for the STARR procedure in Obstructed Defecation Syndrome: Position statement of the group of STARR Pioneers. *Surgical Innovation*, 15: 105-109.

Sielaff M., Scherer R., Gogler H. & Farke S. (2006). Die STARR-Operation. Erfahrungen bei 60 Patienten. *Coloproctology,* 28: 217-223.

Siproudhis L., Ropert A., Lucas J., Raoul J.-L., Heresbach D., Bretagne J.-F. & Gosselin M. (1992). Defecatory disorders, anorectal and pelvic floor dysfunction: A polygamy? *International Journal of Colorectal Disease,* 7: 102-107.

Appendices

List of key words

Titles available

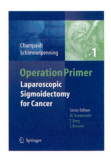 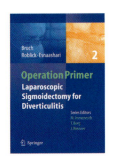 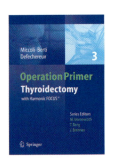 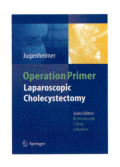 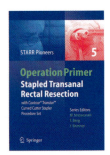

Volume 1: Laparoscopic Sigmoidectomy for Cancer   ISBN 978-3-540-78453-1

Volume 2: Laparoscopic Sigmoidectomy for Diverticulitis   ISBN 978-3-540-78451-7

Volume 3: Thyroidectomy with Harmonic FOCUS®   ISBN 978-3-540-85163-9

Volume 4: Laparoscopic Cholecystectomy   ISBN 978-3-540-92961-1

Volume 5: Stapled Transanal Rectal Resection (STARR)
           with Contour® Transtar™ Curved Cutter Stapler Procedure Set   ISBN 978-3-540-92958-1

Titles in preparation

Laparoscopic Total Mesorectal Excision (TME) for Cancer

Laparoscopic Gastric Banding with the Swedish Adjustable Gastric Band (SAGB VC)

Open Rectal Resection

Laparoscopic Gastric Bypass

Printing and Binding: Stürtz GmbH, Würzburg